PACE The PANCE

PA Review Series

Pediatrics End of Rotation Exam

E. ROMAN

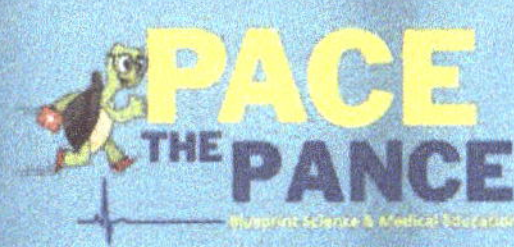

Name: Eric A. Roman, author.
Title: PACE The PANCE PA Review Series Pediatrics End of Rotation Exam
Identifiers: ISBN 978-1-312-36063-1
Imprint: Lulu.com

Before proceeding with the use of any medical book or resource, it is essential to acknowledge and understand the following advisory warning. By accessing or utilizing the information provided within this medical book, you agree to accept full responsibility for any decisions made and the outcomes that may result. It is strongly recommended to consult with qualified healthcare professionals and exercise caution when applying any medical knowledge acquired from this book.

No Medical Advice: The content within this medical book, including texts, illustrations, diagrams, and any accompanying materials, is for informational purposes only. It is not intended to be a substitute for professional medical advice, diagnosis, or treatment. Always seek the guidance of qualified healthcare providers regarding any medical conditions, treatments, or concerns.

Individual Variations: Every individual is unique, and medical conditions may vary significantly from person to person. The information provided in this medical book is general in nature and may not be applicable or suitable for everyone. Exercise caution when interpreting and applying the information to your specific circumstances.

Potential Inaccuracies: The work provided here is "as is." Despite diligent efforts to ensure accuracy and up-to-date information, medical knowledge is constantly evolving. There may be errors, omissions, or discrepancies in the content of this medical book. Therefore, the author, publisher, and associated parties cannot guarantee the completeness, accuracy, or reliability of the information presented herein.

Risks and Consequences: Any medical intervention or decision carries inherent risks. The author, publisher, and associated parties disclaim any and all liability for any direct, indirect, or consequential losses, damages, or injuries that may arise from the application of information contained in this medical book. It is essential to weigh the benefits, risks, and potential consequences before implementing any medical advice or procedures.

Personal Responsibility: By utilizing this medical book, you acknowledge and accept that you are solely responsible for your choices, actions, and outcomes. The author, publisher, and associated parties cannot be held liable for any adverse results or unfavorable experiences that may occur due to the use or misuse of the information presented herein.

Consultation with Healthcare Professionals: It is strongly advised to consult with qualified healthcare professionals, such as doctors, nurses, or specialists, before making any medical decisions. These professionals possess the necessary expertise and experience to provide personalized advice and address individual medical needs effectively. Remember, medical knowledge and understanding are dynamic fields, and advancements occur continuously. Stay informed about the latest research and consult trusted healthcare professionals to make informed decisions regarding your health and well-being. By proceeding further, you indicate that you have read, understood, and agreed to the terms and conditions outlined in this advisory warning. To the maximum extent permitted under the law, no responsibility shall be assumed by the publisher for any and all injury and or damage to persons or property as a matter of products liability, negligence law or otherwise, from any reference to or use by any persons of this work.

To my incredible friends and loving family who have supported me endlessly.

To my clinical preceptors who helped me build my foundation of clinical medicine.

To my alma mater, UC Davis, Johns Hopkins, and USC and all of the faculty and staff who supported me in my academic journey to reach this point in my academic career.

(Page intentionally left blank for students to leave notes here)

About the Author

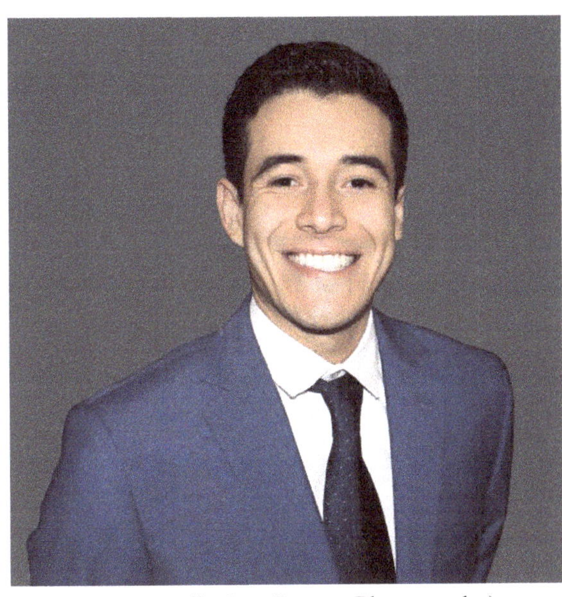

(Photo credit: Ray Roman Photography)

Eric A. Roman, M.S., is an author, educator, and a bilingual Physician Assistant (PA) student at Keck School of Medicine of the University of Southern California (USC). He values patient advocacy and service for the homeless and underserved communities of the Greater Los Angeles area. Prior to PA school, he was driven to use his Spanish-speaking skills; he committed to his patients in the San Fernando Valley while working at the Family Rescue Center, connecting low-income patients to primary healthcare resources. Eric has advocated for the uninsured, immigrant, and homeless populations in Sacramento through a student-run clinic, Clinica Tepati, while earning his undergraduate degree in Neurobiology, Physiology, and Behavior and Spanish double major at the University of California at Davis. He then went on to The Johns Hopkins University School of Medicine and earned a Master of Science degree in Anatomy Education. He specialized in medical education and health professions education curriculum development and became an anatomist, a long-term goal of his. Now, he is currently in his third year of PA school at USC on his clinical rotations and expects to graduate in May of 2024. He has conducted intensive research collaborating with researchers from Hopkins and USC and presented his research at the California Academy of Physician Assistants Conference (CAPACon) in 2022. His research elucidated key themes about the potential to enhance anatomy education and PA education research to prepare PA students to become competent clinicians (Roman et al., 2021). He seeks to enhance fellow PA students' comprehension of basic medical sciences, medical education, and clinical skills. As a clinical student, he is not only determined to provide the utmost care to his patients in the clinic, but he is also passionate about educating and spends his free time building resources for PA students that he shares on his PACE The PANCE social media platforms and websites. He hopes to one day build a platform with resources that will help PA students thrive during their didactic and clinical training. In his free time, he enjoys Crossfit, playing the guitar, and spending time with his family.

(Page intentionally left blank for students to leave notes here)

Preface

Learning in PA school is multimodal, fast-paced, and high-stakes. To be successful, you must swiftly find what works for you. Oftentimes in PA school, there will be multiple resources you come across. The best way to navigate your didactic and clinical training is to find a few resources and stick with them. The more you jump around constantly finding new sources, you may find yourself overwhelmed with information overload, unsure of which resources to use. I strongly recommend slowing yourself down, opening a paper resource, and writing down concepts on a whiteboard or blank piece of paper. In our era of digital consumption, we find ourselves constantly in front of a computer screen (or iPhone, iPad, or other digital devices). We must find a way to connect on a deeper level with the information and I have found from my training in PA school that unplugging from social media, online resources, and computer screens creates a more manageable, comprehensive, and fundamental recipe for understanding the basic medical concepts you need to be successful on your didactic exams and clinical shelf exams.

I have always been a life-long learner. My journey to educating began notably in 2017 when I started to tutor students in organic chemistry. It became a passion, a commitment, and dedication to helping others achieve their goals. To this day, I still tutor students in organic chemistry. Not only that, but I also tutor students in biochemistry, cell biology, physiology, anatomy, Medical College Admission Test (MCAT) content, Poast-Baccalaureate (Post-Bacc) courses, medical sciences, and now, Physician Assistant National Certifying Exam (PANCE) review content. I have a luster for teaching, mentoring, building; I am a content creator and I hope my passion for educating comes through in this book that I have created for PA students who will traverse the same set of circumstances put before them that I had to overcome.

Formula for success on your end of rotation (EOR) exams can be described in the following: 1) recognize the disease that is presented to you in a clinical vignette. 2) decide the workup and management you would like to conduct for your patient that is timely, cost-effective, accurate, and that will provide evidence-based care to alleviate the patients of their signs and symptoms they are experiencing.

This book is unique in the sense that the information can be reached at the tips of your fingers in a timely fashion. Each disease state matches the blueprint content that the National Commission on Certification of Physician Assistants (NCCPA) has posted on their website for PA students who will be taking their EOR exams. By carefully covering each disease state found on the blueprint, this book is comprehensive covering definition, signs and symptoms, etiology, risk factors, labs, imaging, diagnosis, treatment, health maintenance, patient education, and more. There are high-yield facts for each disease state. There are clinical vignettes woven throughout the book to provide ample opportunities to test your knowledge. Each question is carefully crafted with the intention of testing the most common presentations seen on exams.

For viewer pleasure, the set-up of this book is simple: 2 columns with questions on the left and answers on the right. This will quickly help you test your knowledge on-the-spot and give you an opportunity to cover the answers on the right and attempt to recall the answers before revealing them. Once again, these questions follow the blueprint for your EORs and are in alphabetical order divided by appropriate chapters covering each body system (e.g., Cardiology, Dermatology, EENT, etc).

Finally, at the conclusion of this book, you will find a 50 question MCQ practice EOR mock exam to test your wits and knowledge of the content for your Pediatric EOR. New editions can be introduced with constructive feedback provided. We hope you enjoy the contents of this book!

(Page intentionally left blank for students to leave notes here)

TABLE OF CONTENTS

- Hand-foot-and-mouth disease
- Herpes simplex
- Influenza
- Measles
- Mumps
- Pertussis
- Pinworms
- Roseola
- Rubella
- Varicella infection

- Acute rheumatic fever
- Atrial septal defect
- Coarctation of the aorta
- Hypertrophic cardiomyopathy
- Kawasaki disease
- Patent ductus arteriosus
- Syncope
- Tetralogy of Fallot
- Ventricular septal defect

- Appendicitis
- Colic
- Constipation
- Dehydration
- Duodenal atresia
- Encopresis
- Foreign body
- Gastroenteritis
- Gastroesophageal reflux disease
- Hepatitis
- Hirschsprung disease
- Inguinal hernia
- Intussusception
- Jaundice
- Lactose intolerance
- Niacin deficiencies
- Pyloric stenosis
- Umbilical hernia
- Vitamin A deficiency
- Vitamin C deficiency
- Vitamin D deficiency

- Anticipatory guidance
- Down syndrome
- Febrile seizure
- Immunization guidelines
- Meningitis
- Normal growth and development
- Seizure disorders
- Teething
- Turner syndrome

ACNE VULGARIS

What is the pathophysiology of acne vulgaris?	Increased levels of androgens -> inflammation of pilosebaceous units -> increased sebum production due to hormonal stimulation and accumulating keratin debris leads to blockage of pilosebaceous units. Cutibacterium acnes can proliferate -> lead to papules, pustules, nodules, and/or cysts
What is the initial treatment for acne vulgaris? If severe or refractory, what other treatment options are there?	Topical benzoyl peroxide Significant acne that causes psychological stress—tetracycline (e.g., doxycycline). Then—oral isotretinoin (category X, obtain 2 negative pregnancy tests prior to initiation)

ANDROGENIC ALOPECIA

What is the most common cause of hair loss in women?	Androgenic alopecia
Which hormones can influence androgenic alopecia?	Androgenic alopecia is influenced by hormones, particularly androgens such as dihydrotestosterone (DHT). Increased levels of DHT can cause the hair follicles to shrink, leading to shorter and finer hair growth.
What is the treatment for androgenic alopecia?	Minoxidil/Rogaine. Other options: finasteride, spironolactone
What is the pathognomonic finding for alopecia areata?	Exclamation point hairs

ATOPIC DERMATITIS

What is a synonymous term to describe atopic dermatitis?	Eczema
Atopic dermatitis is often associated with which other diseases?	Other atopic diseases (e.g., asthma or allergic rhinitis)
What are the signs and symptoms of atopic dermatitis?	Pruritis, dry skin, eczema of face, head, extensor surfaces and diaper area (infants), flexural creases (children), antecubital fossa; lichenification of the flexor surfaces
What is the treatment for atopic dermatitis?	Avoid triggers, moisturize skin, topical emollients. First-line: topical steroids, 2nd line: topical calcineurin inhibitors. Others: antihistamine (e.g., hydroxyzine or Benadryl). PUVA phototherapy
Which medications can specifically help with pruritis?	Benadryl, Zyrtec or Allegra
What is the atopic triad?	Asthma, allergic rhinitis, and atopic dermatitis

BURNS

What is the name of the formula commonly used to determine the amount of fluid resuscitation needed within 24 hours of sustaining a significant burn?	Parkland formula

A first-degree burn involves only which layer of skin?	Epidermis only
A second-degree superficial partial thickness burn involves which layers of skin?	Epidermis and superficial dermis
A second-degree deep partial thickness burn involves which layers of skin?	Epidermis, superficial dermis, and deep dermis
A third-degree burn involves which layers of skin?	Epidermis, dermis, and subcutaneous fat
A fourth-degree burn involves which layers of skin?	Epidermis, dermis, subcutaneous fat, and deeper structures (e.g., muscle, fascia, fat, bone)

DERMATITIS

What is the most common etiology for diaper dermatitis?	Candida albicans
Which laboratory test can confirm the diagnosis of candidal dermatitis?	KOH prep
Treatment of choice for candida dermatitis?	Topical antifungal (e.g., nystatin)
What is the treatment for diaper dermatitis with satellite lesions?	Petroleum jelly, zinc oxide (Desitin), and nystatin
Perioral dermatitis spares which anatomical location?	Vermillion border of the lip margin
Initial treatment of choice for perioral dermatitis?	Topical metronidazole

SEBORRHEIC DERMATITIS

What is seborrheic dermatitis?	Common chronic inflammatory condition that affects the scalp
What is the pathophysiology of seborrheic dermatitis?	Over-secretion of sebaceous contents; colonization of yeast
What is the etiology of seborrheic dermatitis?	Malassezia furfur yeast
What are the signs and symptoms for seborrheic dermatitis?	**Greasy-yellow**, scaly rash with erythematous plaques and scaly patches on the scalp. Can also affect ears, eyebrows, chest, and groinW
What is the treatment for seborrheic dermatitis?	Emollients, mineral oil, creams or shampoos containing selenium sulfide, zinc pyrithione, salicylic acid; ketoconazole (antifungal, first line therapy), topical corticosteroids for acute flares. For severe cases or refractory—oral ketoconazole or fluconazole

DRUG ERUPTIONS

A 3-year-old boy presents to the pediatrician for a follow appointment after recently diagnosed and treated for acute otitis media. On exam, his tympanic membranes are clear. His chest is notable for a non-pruritic erythematous rash that covers his thoracic cavity and upper extremities bilaterally. Which agent likely caused this condition based on his previous medical history?	Amoxicillin; an adverse reaction can occur in response to the course of amoxicillin for his recently diagnosed acute otitis media
An 18-year-old girl was recently diagnosed with acute pyelonephritis. She was given an IM injection of ceftriaxone and prescribed oral ciprofloxacin for management. Two hours later she returned to clinic with an itchy rash. On exam, she has well-circumscribed papules on an erythematous base. What is the name of this acute condition in which she developed?	Acute urticaria via an IgE-mediated mast cell activation (type 1 hypersensitivity). This can occur in response to beta lactams (e.g., PCN) and cephalosporins (e.g., ceftriaxone)

What are 2 very common drug reactions?	1) Stevens-Johnson Syndrome is a severe, life-threatening drug reaction characterized by a widespread skin rash, blistering, and mucosal involvement. It is often caused by certain medications, such as antibiotics (e.g., sulfonamides) and antiepileptic drugs (e.g., phenytoin). 2) Toxic Epidermal Necrolysis is a severe and rare drug reaction that involves extensive detachment of the epidermis, resembling a severe burn. It is often triggered by medications, including sulfonamides, anticonvulsants, and nonsteroidal anti-inflammatory drugs (NSAIDs).
What is DRESS syndrome?	Drug Rash with Eosinophilia and Systemic Symptoms, also known as DRESS syndrome, is a severe hypersensitivity reaction characterized by rash, fever, lymphadenopathy, and involvement of internal organs (e.g., liver, kidney). Antiepileptic drugs and allopurinol are common culprits.

ERYTHEMA MULTIFORME

Which type of hypersensitivity reaction occurs in erythema multiforme?	Type IV hypersensitivity reaction
Most common etiology for erythema multiforme?	HSV
Other causes of erythema multiforme?	PCN, sulfonamides, barbiturates, phenytoin
Describe the physical exam findings of erythema multiforme.	Central erythematous lesion surrounded by a pale edematous ring
(+) or (-) Nikolsky sign in erythema multiforme?	(-) Nikolsky sign
Describe a (+) Nikolsky sign based on physical exam.	Upon light pressure, there is epidermal detachment
Which conditions do you see a (+) Nikolsky sign?	Toxic epidermal detachment (TEN), Steven-Johnson Syndrome (SJS), and pemphigus vulgaris

EXANTHEMS

FIFTH DISEASE

What is another name for Fifth disease?	Erythema infectiosum
What is the most common cause of Fifth disease?	Parvovirus B19
What is the classic skin manifestation that occurs in Fifth disease?	Macular slapped-cheek appearance rash on face

HAND-FOOT-MOUTH DISEASE

What is hand-foot-mouth disease?	Childhood infection that produces sores/vesicles of the pharynx as well as an erythematous rash about the hands, feet, and buttocks
What is the etiology of hand-foot-mouth disease?	Coxsackievirus A16
Which age group is most likely to develop hand-foot-mouth disease?	< 5 years old
Most likely mechanism of transmission for hand-foot-mouth disease?	Person-person contact, respiratory droplets
What signs and symptoms are present with hand-foot-mouth disease?	Rash, vesiculo-ulcerative lesions of the pharynx, and fever, sore throat, irritability, and loss of appetite
What is the treatment for hand-foot-mouth disease?	Supportive care; the virus is self-limiting. Can offer pain medications for painful ulcerative lesions. Acetaminophen for fevers prn

MEASLES

What is the other name for Measles?	Rubeola

What are the 3 C's of measles?	Cough, coryza, and conjunctivitis
What is the pathognomonic finding for measles on physical exam?	Koplik spots
What are Koplik spots?	Bluish white macules on the buccal mucosa
What is the name of the virus responsible for measles?	Paramyxovirus
Is the measles virus RNA or DNA?	Single stranded RNA virus
Which vitamin can be given to patients hospitalized with measles?	Vitamin A can decrease morbidity and mortality
What is the only way to prevent measles?	Vaccination
What is the name of the vaccine given to patients?	MMR vaccine
What is the vaccine schedule for the MMR vaccine?	12 months and 4 years of age
In which direction is the rash spread in the development of measles?	Cephalocaudal spread (e.g., spread from head to extremities)
Name two complications that occur due to measles?	Encephalitis and pneumonia

What is another name for Rubella?	German measles
In which direction is the rash spread in the development of measles?	Cephalocaudal spread (e.g., spread from head to extremities)
Which lymph nodes develop lymphadenopathy in Rubella?	Posterior cervical and posterior auricular lymphadenopathy
How do you differentiate Rubella from Rubeola?	Rubella rash spreads much more rapidly and does not coalesce
Treatment for Rubella?	Supportive care
What is the only way to prevent Rubella?	Vaccination
Congenital Rubella can cause what manifestations?	Sensorineural hearing loss, intellectual impairment, cardiovascular and ocular defects

What is the etiology of Roseola?	HHV-6
Signs and symptoms of Roseola?	High fever followed by erythematous rash on trunk that spreads to extremities and face
How is Roseola transmitted?	Roseola is primarily spread through respiratory secretions, such as coughing and sneezing. It can also be transmitted through close contact with an infected person
How is Roseola diagnosed?	Roseola is usually diagnosed based on the characteristic symptoms and physical examination. In some cases, blood tests may be done to confirm the presence of the virus.
What is the treatment for Roseola?	Self-resolving
How long does Roseola last?	The fever associated with Roseola usually lasts for about 3 to 5 days, while the rash typically appears after the fever subsides and lasts for 1 to 2 days.

What is the most common cause of impetigo?	Staph aureus or strep pyogenes
What is the most common age group for impetigo?	Ages 2-6 years old
What are the signs and symptoms of impetigo?	Signs and symptoms of impetigo include red sores or blisters that quickly rupture, oozing a fluid that forms a characteristic honey-colored crust. It may be itchy and can occur anywhere on the body, but commonly affects the face, hands, and diaper area in children.

What is the best non-pharmacological treatment for impetigo?	Non-pharmacological treatment for impetigo includes gentle cleansing of the affected areas with soap and water to remove crusts and prevent the spread of infection. Good hygiene practices, such as frequent handwashing, are important to minimize the risk of transmission.
What is the best initial pharmacological treatment for a patient diagnosed with impetigo?	Topical mupirocin

MOLLUSCUM CONTAGIOSUM

What is molluscum contagiosum?	Molluscum contagiosum is a viral skin infection characterized by small, flesh-colored bumps on the skin's surface.
What is the name of the virus that causes molluscum contagiosum?	Poxvirus
What are the signs and symptoms of molluscum contagiosum?	Small, flesh-colored bumps on the skin that may be itchy or inflamed.
What is the treatment for molluscum contagiosum?	Non-pharmacological treatment may include cryotherapy, curettage, or laser therapy to remove the lesions. Pharmacological treatments include topical medications like imiquimod or cantharidin that can be applied directly to the lesions.

LICE

What are the 3 types of lice?	Lice infestations are caused by three types of lice: head lice (Pediculus humanus capitis), body lice (Pediculus humanus corporis), and pubic lice (Pthirus pubis). They spread through direct contact with infested individuals or sharing personal items like combs, hats, or clothing.
What is the most common type of lice?	Head lice (Pediculus humanus capitis) are the most common type of lice infestation.
What are the signs and symptoms of lice?	Lice infestation include scalp itching, visible lice or nits (lice eggs) attached to hair shafts, small red bumps or sores on the scalp, and presence of lice or nits on personal items like combs or clothing.
How do lice infestations spread? **a) Through airborne transmission** **b) By consuming contaminated food** **c) Via direct contact or sharing personal items** **d) Through exposure to infected animals**	Answer: C) via direct contact or sharing personal items
How is the diagnosis of lice infestation typically made? **a) Blood test** **b) Skin biopsy** **c) Finding live lice or nits in the hair or scalp** **d) Imaging tests**	Answer: c) Finding live lice or nits in the hair or scalp
What is the drug of choice for lice?	Permethrin

LICHEN PLANUS

What is lichen planus?	Lichen planus is an autoimmune skin condition characterized by itchy, flat-topped papules with a polygonal shape.
What are the 5 P's of lichen planus?	Pruritic, purple, polygonal, planar, papules

What are the common clinical features of lichen planus?
a) Itchy, flat-topped papules with a polygonal shape
b) Vesicles and bullae on the skin
c) Excessive hair growth in affected areas
d) Smooth, shiny patches of skin

Answer: a) Itchy, flat-topped papules with a polygonal shape

What is the recommended non-pharmacological treatment for lichen planus?
a) Application of topical corticosteroids
b) Ultraviolet (UV) light therapy
c) Oral antihistamines
d) Regular moisturizing of the affected areas

Answer: d) Regular moisturizing of the affected areas

Which medication is commonly prescribed for severe or widespread lichen planus?
a) Oral corticosteroids
b) Antibiotics
c) Antifungal creams
d) Topical retinoids

Answer: a) Oral corticosteroids
Explanation: topical steroids can be used initially; second line therapy is systemic steroids. Retinoids, abx, or fungal meds are not indicated

PEDICULOSIS

What is pediculosis?
a) Fungal skin infection
b) Viral skin infection
c) Bacterial skin infection
d) Parasitic infestation

Answer: d) Parasitic infestation

What is pediculosis capitis?

Head lice

What are common signs and symptoms of lice infestation?
a) Intense scalp itching
b) Visible lice or nits (lice eggs)
c) Small red bumps or sores on the scalp
d) All of the above

Answer: d) All of the above

What is the treatment for pediculosis capitis?

Permethrin 1% shampoo

PITYRIASIS ROSEA

What is pityriasis rosea?

Pityriasis rosea is a common, self-limited skin condition characterized by an initial herald patch followed by the appearance of smaller, pink or salmon-colored oval-shaped patches on the trunk and limbs.

What is the etiology of pityriasis rosea?

The exact cause of pityriasis rosea is unknown, but it is believed to be associated with viral infections, particularly the human herpesvirus 6 (HHV-6) and HHV-7.

What are the characteristic signs and symptoms of pityriasis rosea?
a) Small, itchy blisters on the hands and feet
b) Red, scaly patches on the scalp
c) Pink or salmon-colored oval-shaped patches on the trunk and limbs
d) Raised, silver-colored plaques on the elbows and knees

Answer: c) Pink or salmon-colored oval-shaped patches on the trunk and limbs

What is the characteristic pattern called that is found on the trunk? (hint: not herald patch)

Christmas tree pattern

What is the treatment for pityriasis rosea?

There is no specific pharmacological treatment for pityriasis rosea. However, if itching is severe, topical corticosteroids or antihistamines may be prescribed for symptomatic relief.

SCABIES

What is scabies?	Scabies is a highly contagious parasitic infestation of the skin caused by the Sarcoptes scabiei mite.
What are the typical signs and symptoms of scabies? **a) Itchy, raised, red bumps or blisters on the skin** **b) Dry, scaly patches on the scalp** **c) Painful, pus-filled sores on the hands and feet** **d) Yellow discoloration of the skin**	Answer: a) Itchy, raised, red bumps or blisters on the skin
What findings are expected during the history and physical examination for scabies?	Intense pruritis especially at night. Physical examination may reveal characteristic skin lesions, burrows, and excoriations, especially in the web spaces between the fingers, wrists, elbows, and genital areas.
What is the treatment for scabies?	Topical permethrin cream or oral ivermectin if extensive involvement. These medications kill the mites and their eggs.

STEVEN-JOHNSON SYNDROME (SJS)

What is SJS?	Immune-mediated skin reaction -> blistering of the skin and epidermal detachment
SJS is which percentage of epidermal detachment?	< 10%
What are common triggers of SJS?	Drugs (e.g., antibiotics—sulfonamides, aminopenicillins, rifampin; corticosteroids, antiepileptics, allopurinol, sulfasalazine), infections, idiopathic
What are the signs and symptoms of SJS?	Fever, malaise, sore throat, myalgia, arthralgia, mucocutaneous lesions, lesions form bullae/vesicles
(+) or (-) Nikolsky sign in SJS?	(+) Nikolsky sign, extensive epidermal necrosis and sloughing
What is the percentage of epidermal detachment for SJS/TEN?	Between 10-30%

TOXIC EPIDERMAL NECROLYSIS (TEN)

What is the epidermal detachment percentage for TEN?	>30%
What are drugs that can trigger TEN?	Sulfonamides, allopurinol, NSAIDs, phenobarbital, carbamazepine, and lamotrigine
What is the treatment for SJS/TEN?	Discontinue any offending agents, IV fluids, parenteral nutrition, IV pain meds, wound care, treat severe burns, continued fluid and electrolyte replacement

TINEA

What is tinea?	Fungal skin infections of the keratinized tissues (e.g., skin, nails, hair)
What is the best diagnostic test for tinea?	KOH prep
What is tinea capitis?	Infection of the scalp hair
Tinea capitis is most commonly caused by what etiology?	*Trichophyton tonsurans*
What is the term to describe a painful mass/loose hair on the scalp characterized by inflammatory plaques with pustules and thick crusting?	Kerion
What is the treatment of choice for tinea capitis?	Oral Giseofulvin

What is tinea barbae?	Papules/pustules of the hair follicles of the beard in males
What is tinea unguium?	Dermatophyte onychomycosis—aka fungal infection of the nail
What is tinea pedis?	Athlete's foot
What is the most common dermatophyte infection?	Tinea pedis (athlete's foot)
What is tinea cruris?	"Jock itch"
What is the treatment for tinea cruris?	Topical antifungal (e.g., Ketoconazole, econazole, etc.)
What is the tinea corporis?	Ring worm
What is the first line treatment for tinea corporis?	Topical antifungal Then, oral Terbinafine
Tinea versicolor is most commonly caused by what etiology?	*Malassezia furfur*
What is the most common finding on KOH prep for tinea versicolor?	Spaghetti and meatballs (e.g., short hyphae and clusters of spores)
What is the treatment for tinea versicolor?	Selenium sulfide or zinc pyrithione; topical antifungal Systemic therapy: oral itraconazole or fluconazole if widespread and failed topical therapy

Urticaria is also called what?	Hives
How would you describe the physical exam findings of urticaria?	Pruritic, well-circumscribed erythematous plaques (e.g., wheals)
Urticaria is due to which type of cells?	Mast cell activation
What is the treatment for urticaria?	H1 + H2 + steroid (e.g., prednisolone 20-50 mg/day x 10 days) If anaphylaxis present, give epinephrine If chronic, give second-generation antihistamine H1 blockers (e.g., Claritin, Allegra)

What is the cause of verrucae?	HPV
What are the 3 types of verrucae?	Verruca vulgaris (common) Verruca plantaris (plantar) Verruca plana (flat warts)
What is the pathognomonic finding for verrucae?	Common and plantar warts- thrombosed capillaries red-brown punctuations)
Condyloma acuminatum is due to which types of HPV?	HPV 6 and 11
What is the treatment for verrucae?	Most self-resolve within 2 years, can perform cryotherapy with liquid nitrogen; or can offer self-administered salicylic acid

ACUTE OTITIS MEDIA

What are four causes of acute otitis media?	Streptococcus pneumoniae, Haemophilus influenzae, Moraxella catarrhalis, and strep pyogenes
What is the most the following is the most common cause of acute otitis media?	Streptococcus pneumoniae
What are the signs and symptoms of acute otitis media?	Bulging TM, reduced mobility, erythema
What is the treatment of acute otitis media?	High dose amoxicillin is first line. If recurrent, can give Augmentin. If allergy, can give cephalosporin. If severe, can give doxycycline or macrolide
What is one complication of acute otitis media?	Mastoiditis

ACUTE PHARYNGOTONSILLITIS

What is the most common cause of acute pharyngotonsillitis?	Adenovirus
What is the most common etiology for strep pharyngitis?	Group A beta-hemolytic streptococci
What is the name of the criteria to diagnose strep pharyngitis?	Centor criteria
What makes up the Centor criteria?	Absence of cough, exudates on tonsils, fever, and anterior cervical lymphadenopathy
What is the gold standard for diagnosing strep pharyngitis?	Throat culture
What is the first line treatment for group A strep?	Penicillin
What is the treatment for group A strep for a patient with a penicillin allergy?	Azithromycin
List two complications of group A strep?	Rheumatic fever and post-strep glomerulonephritis

MONONUCLEOSIS

What is the etiology of mononucleosis?	Mononucleosis is primarily caused by the Epstein-Barr virus (EBV), although other viruses such as cytomegalovirus (CMV) can also cause similar symptoms.
What are the most common modes of transmission of mononucleosis?	Mononucleosis is typically transmitted through direct contact with the saliva of an infected person, such as kissing or sharing utensils.
What are the typical signs and symptoms of mononucleosis? **a) Cough, runny nose, and sore throat** **b) Rash, joint pain, and muscle weakness** **c) Fatigue, sore throat, swollen lymph nodes, and fever** **d) Headache, nausea, and abdominal pain**	Answer: c) Fatigue, sore throat, swollen lymph nodes, and fever
What findings are expected during the physical examination for mononucleosis? **a) Enlarged liver and yellowing of the skin** **b) Rash and joint swelling** **c) Rapid breathing and wheezing** **d) Enlarged lymph nodes and a red throat**	Answer: d) Enlarged lymph nodes and a red throat

What is the name of the test to diagnose mononucleosis?	Heterophile agglutination test (monospot)
What is the recommended treatment for confirmed mononucleosis? **a) Bed rest and adequate hydration** **b) Regular exercise and a balanced diet** **c) Topical creams for symptom relief** **d) Antibiotics to target the causative virus**	Answer: a) Bed rest and adequate hydration Mono is due to EBV virus, so antibiotic therapy is not indicated.
What is one important patient education piece to share with athletic adolescents diagnosed with mononucleosis?	Refrain from contact sports for 3-4 weeks (due to splenomegaly and increased risk of splenic a. bleeding)

What are signs and symptoms of allergic rhinitis?	Clear rhinorrhea, sneezing, water eyes, itchy eyes, clear nasal discharge
What are common physical exam findings you may discover on physical exam?	Allergic shiners (blue discoloration below the eyes), turbinates edematous and pale
What is the recommended non-pharmacological treatment for allergic rhinitis? **a) Antihistamine medications** **b) Nasal corticosteroid sprays** **c) Avoidance of allergens, such as using dust mite covers and keeping windows closed** **d) Decongestant medications**	Answer: c) Avoidance of allergens, such as using dust mite covers and keeping windows closed
What is the recommended pharmacological treatment for allergic rhinitis? **a) Antibiotics to target underlying bacterial infection** **b) Antifungal medications for fungal-related rhinitis** **c) Antiviral medications for viral-related rhinitis** **d) Antihistamine medications and nasal corticosteroid sprays**	Answer: d) Antihistamine medications and nasal corticosteroid sprays
What are examples of medications typically used for allergic rhinitis?	Claritin (or Zyrtec) and flonase
What is an important aspect of patient education for allergic rhinitis?	Patient education should focus on understanding triggers, implementing allergen avoidance measures, and discussing the benefits of long-term management options such as allergy shots or immunotherapy.

What is the treatment of allergic conjunctivitis?	Allergen avoidance, cold compress, topical antihistamines. Oral antihistamines
What is the most common cause of viral conjunctivitis?	Adenovirus
What is one finding on physical exam you may find in the workup of viral conjunctivitis? Eyes "glued shut" in the mornings **A) Cobblestone mucosa of the posterior oropharynx** **B) Course crackles on auscultation** **C) Preauricular lymphadenopathy** **D) Pruritus**	C) Preauricular lymphadenopathy You are likely to find preauricular lymphadenopathy on physical exam in the workup of viral conjunctivitis. Eyes "glued shut" in the mornings is likely to be bacterial conjunctivitis. Cobblestone mucosa of the posterior oropharynx is characteristic of allergic conjunctivitis. Course crackles on auscultation is worrisome for potential pneumonia. Pruritis is more characteristic for allergic conjunctivitis

| What is the most common cause of bacterial conjunctivitis among contact lens users? | Pseudomonas aeruginosa |
| What is the treatment for bacterial conjunctivitis? | Erythromycin ointment |

What is epiglottitis?	Supraglottic inflammation of the airway
What is the etiology of epiglottitis?	Haemophilus influenzae type B
What are the 3 D's of epiglottitis?	Dysphagia, drooling, and respiratory distress
What are the signs and symptoms of epiglottitis?	Dysphagia, drooling, respiratory distress, inspiratory stridor, cough, fever, restlessness
How will patients with epiglottitis position themselves?	Tripod position—sitting, leaning forward, elbows braced, chin thrust forward, and neck hyperextended
Which x-ray should be ordered in the work up of epiglottitis?	Lateral cervical radiograph
What is the classic x-ray finding in the diagnosis of epiglottitis?	Thumbprint sign
What is the definitive way to diagnose epiglottitis?	Laryngoscopy
What is the treatment of epiglottitis?	Secure airway, dexamethasone to decrease inflammation, consider intubation, antibiotics (e.g., ceftriaxone or cefotaxime)

Which nose bleed is more common, anterior or posterior?	Anterior nosebleed
What is the most common cause of anterior epistaxis?	Trauma
Which of the following arteries is responsible for posterior epistaxis? A) Kisselbach plexus B) Facial artery C) Maxillary artery D) Sphenopalatine artery E) Inferior alveolar artery	D) Sphenopalatine artery
What is the Kisselbach plexus?	Kisselbach plexus is a region in the anterior part of the nasal septum where several blood vessels converge, making it a common site for nosebleeds.
What is the treatment for a posterior epistaxis?	Posterior balloon packing
What are the non-pharmacological and pharmacological treatment options for epistaxis?	Non-pharmacological treatment includes applying direct pressure to the nose, leaning forward slightly, and keeping the nasal passages moist with saline sprays. Pharmacological treatment may involve the use of nasal decongestants, topical antibiotics, or cauterization procedures for severe or recurrent cases.

Classifications of hearing impairment?	Conductive, sensorineural or both
What is the most common cause of conductive hearing loss?	Cerumen impaction followed by acute otitis media
What is the most common cause of sensorineural hearing loss?	Presbycusis
What is the main treatment option for sensorineural hearing impairment? a) Medications to restore hearing b) Hearing aids c) Surgery to repair the inner ear	Answer: b) Hearing aids

d) Antibiotics to treat infections

MASTOIDITIS

Mastoiditis occurs as a complication of which disease?	Acute otitis media
Signs and symptoms of mastoiditis?	Deep ear pain worse at night, fever, lethargy, mastoid tenderness, protrusion of the auricle
What kind of imaging will you order for the diagnosis of mastoiditis?	CT scan with contrast; or MRI is highly sensitive
What is the treatment of mastoiditis?	IV antibiotics (e.g., ceftriaxone)

ORAL CANDIDIASIS

Oral candidiasis is also called what?	Oral thrush
What is the etiology of oral thrush?	Candida albicans
What is the name of the smear to diagnose oral candidiasis?	KOH smear
What is the treatment for oral thrush?	Nystatin

ORBITAL CELLULITIS

What is orbital cellulitis?	Infection of the orbital muscles and fat posteriorly to the eye
What is one pertinent physical exam finding in the diagnosis of orbital cellulitis?	Decreased extraocular eye movements
How do you diagnose orbital cellulitis?	CT scan of the orbit is confirmatory
What is the treatment for orbital cellulitis?	Hospitalization and IV broad spectrum antibiotics (e.g., vancomycin)

OTITIS EXTERNA

What is another name for otitis externa?	"Swimmer's ear"
What is the classic risk factor for the development of otitis externa?	Swimming or water exposure
What are the signs and symptoms of otitis externa?	Pruritis, discharge, pain with manipulation of the auricle
What is the etiology of otitis externa?	Pseudomonas aeruginosa
What is the treatment for otitis externa?	Antibiotic drops such as fluoroquinolone (e.g., Ciprodex)
When should you seek medical attention for otitis externa? **a) If symptoms worsen or persist despite treatment** **b) If there is severe pain or fever** **c) If there is drainage from the ear** **d) All of the above**	Answer: d) All of the above

PERITONSILLAR ABSCESS

What are the signs and symptoms of peritonsillar abscess?	Sore throat, dysphagia, deviation of the uvula, muffled "hot potato" voice, trismus, halitosis
What typically precedes a peritonsillar abscess?	Tonsillitis or pharyngitis
What is the most common cause of peritonsillar abscess?	Streptococcus pyogenes
What are other etiologies for peritonsillar abscess?	Staph aureus, group A strep, H. flu
Which imaging do you order in the work up a peritonsillar abscess?	X-ray, CT with contrast, or u/s of the neck

| **What is the treatment for peritonsillar abscess?** | Airway management, empiric antibiotics, abscess drainage |

STRABISMUS	
What is strabismus?	Abnormal alignment of the eyes
Which physical exam can detect strabismus?	The cover/uncover test

TYMPANIC MEMBRANE PERFORATION	
Signs and symptoms of tympanic membrane perforation?	Pain, otorrhea, hearing reduction/hearing loss
What is the treatment of tympanic membrane perforation?	Self-resolving, keep dry, surgical repair if persistent *NOTE: consider oral amoxicillin in the setting of acute otitis media leading to the complication of tympanic membrane perforation*

CHAPTER 3 | PULMONOLOGY (12%)

What is the clinical presentation of acute bronchiolitis?	Wheezing, fever, nasal discharge
What is the most common cause of acute bronchiolitis?	RSV
Which populations are most at risk for RSV bronchiolitis?	Infants born before 29 weeks gestation, infants < 32 weeks gestation with a chronic lung disease, infants with congenital heart disease, and children < 24 months who are considered immunocompromised
What is seen on chest x-ray in the diagnosis of acute bronchiolitis?	Often normal, but may show air trapping, hyperinflation, and peri-bronchial thickening
What is the only treatment proven to improve bronchiolitis?	Oxygen
What are the indications for hospitalization?	O2 sat < 95%, toxic-appearing, in acute distress, respiratory distress (e.g., nasal flaring, retractions, RR > 70, cyanosis)

What is the atopic triad?	Eczema, allergic rhinitis, and asthma
Which medications exacerbate asthma?	-Aspirin, NSAIDs, and beta blockers
What is the mainstay of asthma monitoring?	Peak expiratory flow meter
Is asthma reversible or irreversible?	Reversible
What is the mainstay treatment for an acute asthma exacerbation?	Albuterol
What is the dosing?	Albuterol 90 mcg/inh every 4-6 hours as needed
What is a recommended treatment regimen for stepping up the asthma treatment for a patient only using albuterol prn?	ICS/LABA such as budesonide/formoterol (Symbicort)

What is Croup?	Narrowing of the trachea in the subglottic area
What is the most common cause of Croup?	Parainfluenza virus
What is the classic finding for Croup on chest x-ray?	Steeple sign
Croup commonly presents between which ages?	3 months to 5 years old
What is the treatment for croup?	Cool mist humidifier, dexamethasone or prednisolone. If severe (airway likely compromised), give racemic epi (rapidly acting within minutes)

What is the inheritance pattern for cystic fibrosis?	Autosomal recessive
Most common infecting bacteria in cystic fibrosis patients with recurrent pulmonary infections?	Pseudomonas aeruginosa
Which chromosome affected in cystic fibrosis?	Chromosome 7
Which gene is affected in cystic fibrosis?	CFTR gene
What is the pathophysiology of cystic fibrosis?	Dysregulation of chloride transport. Chloride channel responsible for transporting chloride from the lumen into the cell (e.g., reabsorption) is dysfunctional; thus,

there is inability to reabsorb chloride, which also leads to less reabsorption of sodium and water. Results in hyper-viscous mucus

What is seen on chest x-ray in the diagnosis of cystic fibrosis?	Hyperinflation, mucous plugging, and focal atelectasis

FOREIGN BODY

Best way to remove foreign body in pediatric airway?	Rigid open tube bronchoscope
What is the treatment of foreign body aspiration?	Endoscopy

HYALINE MEMBRANE DISEASE

What is the most common cause of hyaline membrane disease?	Deficiency of surfactant
What is the most common cause of respiratory disease in preterm infants?	Hyaline membrane disease
What is seen on chest x-ray in the diagnosis of hyaline membrane disease?	Bilateral diffuse atelectasis -> ground glass appearance
What is the treatment of hyaline membrane disease?	Antenatal steroid within 24-48 hours of birth, mechanical ventilation with positive pressure, endotracheal artificial surfactant, IV fluid replacement

PNEUMONIA

Which pneumonia etiology is suspected in patients with rust-colored sputum?	Strep pneumoniae
Which pneumonia etiology is suspected in patients with currant jelly sputum?	Klebsiella
What is the most common cause of viral pneumonia in children?	RSV
Which physical exam findings are present in acute bacterial pneumonia?	(+) egophony, tactile fremitus, and dullness to percussion
What is the treatment for outpatient bacterial community acquired pneumonia in the pediatric population?	Amoxicillin, amoxicillin-clavulanate, or if severe– macrolide (e.g., azithromycin)
What is the first line therapy for atypical bacteria pneumonia?	Azithromycin. Alternatives–erythromycin or doxycycline

RESPIRATORY SYNCYTIAL VIRUS

Most common cause of lower respiratory tract infection in children worldwide?	RSV
Which population is most at risk for severe RSV infection? a) Infants and young children b) Teenagers and young adults c) Middle-aged adults d) Elderly individuals	Answer: a) Infants and young children
What is the mainstay of treatment for RSV infection? a) Antibiotics b) Antiviral medications c) Supportive care to manage symptoms d) Vaccination	Answer: c) Supportive care to manage symptoms

ATYPICAL MYCOBACTERIAL DISEASE

What is the transmission of mycobacterium avium?	Soil and water
What are the risk factors for mycobacterium avium complex (MAC)?	HIV with CD4 count < 50
What are the clinical manifestations of MAC infection?	Night sweats, fever, weight loss, lymphadenitis, abdominal pain, hepatosplenomegaly
How do you diagnose MAC infection?	Acid fast staining; culture
What is the initial treatment for MAC infection?	At least 2 antimycobacterial medications (e.g., macrolide AND ethambutol)

EPSTEIN-BARR DISEASE

Classic triad for Epstein-Barr mononucleosis?	Fever, lymphadenopathy, and pharyngitis
How do you diagnose Epstein-Barr mononucleosis?	Heterophile antibody screen (Monospot)
What is the transmission for Epstein-Barr mononucleosis?	Respiratory secretions/saliva
What is the treatment for Epstein-Barr mononucleosis?	Symptomatic treatment, self-resolving. Rest, acetaminophen, NSAIDs
What is one classic complication that may result from Epstein-Barr mononucleosis?	Splenomegaly, splenic rupture
What is one patient education piece you would recommend?	Avoid contact sports for three to four weeks

ERYTHEMA INFECTIOSUM

What is another name for erythema infectiosum?	Fifth disease
What is the primary cause of Fifth Disease? a) Bacterial infection b) Fungal infection c) Viral infection d) Parasitic infection	Answer: c) Viral infection
Most common etiology for fifth disease?	Parvovirus B19
What is a classic physical exam finding seen in fifth disease?	Slapped cheek malar rash
What is the treatment for fifth disease?	Supportive, acetaminophen and NSAIDs
How can Fifth Disease be prevented? a) Practicing good hand hygiene b) Avoiding close contact with sick individuals c) Covering the mouth and nose when coughing or sneezing d) All of the above	Answer: d) All of the above

HAND-FOOT-MOUTH DISEASE

What is the etiology for hand-foot-mouth disease?	Coxsackievirus
Which age is most common for the development of hand-foot-mouth disease?	Less than 5 years old
What are the signs and symptoms of hand-foot-mouth disease?	Oral enanthem and a maculopapular rash/vesicular rash on the hands and feet
What is the treatment for hand foot mouth disease?	Self-resolving, pain medications, good hand hygiene

HERPES SIMPLEX

HSV 1 =	Oral lesions
HSV 2 =	Genital lesions
HSV 3 =	Varicella zoster
HSV 4 =	EBV
HSV 5 =	CMV
HSV 6 =	Roseola
HSV 7 =	Not classified
HSV 8 =	Kaposi Sarcoma
Test of choice for herpes simplex-1?	PCR
Gold standard for diagnosing herpes simplex-1?	HSV-1 serology
What is the name of the smear used to identify multinucleated giant cells in patients with HSV?	Tzanck smear
What is the treatment for herpes simplex virus?	Acyclovir

What are the signs and symptoms of influenza?	Fever, coryza, cough, HA, fatigue, malaise, myalgia
How is the diagnosis made for influenza?	Rapid antigen test
What is the gold standard for influenza?	PCR or viral culture
What is the treatment for influenza?	Supportive, self-resolving. If severe, oseltamivir
Measles	
What are the 3 C's of measles?	Cough, coryza, and conjunctivitis
Pathognomonic physical exam finding seen in measles?	Koplik spots
What is the most common cause of measles related deaths?	Pneumonia

What is the name of the virus that causes mumps?	Paramyxovirus
Which gland swelling is associated with mumps?	Parotid gland
When is the first dose of the MMR vaccine given?	12 months of age – 15 months of age
When is the second dose of the MMR vaccine given?	Age 4-6 years
What is the most common complication of mumps?	Orchitis

Pertussis is otherwise known as?	Whooping cough
Pertussis is gram (+) or gram (-)?	Gram (-)
What is the etiology for pertussis?	Bordetella pertussis
What are the three stages of pertussis?	Catarrhal stage, paroxysmal stage, and convalescent stage
What are the signs and symptoms of pertussis?	Rapid-fire coughing followed by inspiratory whoop and post-tussive emesis
When is the DTaP vaccine given?	2 months, 4 months, 6 months, 15-18 months, and ages 4-6 years
What is the treatment for pertussis?	Azithromycin or Bactrim for all household contacts

What is the etiology for pinworms?	Enterobius vermicularis
What is a physical exam test you can do to diagnose pinworms?	Cellophane tape or scotch tape test
What is the treatment for pinworms?	Mebendazole
Rocky mountain spotted fever	
What is the etiology for rocky mountain spotted fever?	Rickettsia rickettsii

What are the signs and symptoms for rocky mountain spotted fever?	Nausea, vomiting, fevers, chills, myalgias, HA, rash (e.g., red maculopapular rash on wrist and ankles)
What is the confirmatory test for rocky mountain spotted fever?	Serologic testing
Treatment of choice for rocky mountain spotted fever in a child?	Doxycycline

What are the signs and symptoms of Roseola?	A high fever for three days followed by a maculopapular rash that starts on the trunk and moves to the face and extremities
What is the pathogen that causes Roseola?	HHV-6
What is the treatment for Roseola?	Supportive, self-resolving. Acetaminophen to lower the fever

What is the other name for Rubella?	German measles
What is the classic triad of congenital rubella?	Patent ductus arteriosus, cataract, and sensorineural hearing loss
What are the signs and symptoms of rubella?	URI prodrome, sub-occipital LAD and posterior auricular LAD, pink nonconfluent maculopapular rash that starts on the face and spreads to trunk and extremities

What is the etiology for scarlet fever?	Streptococcus pyogenes
What are the clinical manifestations of scarlet fever?	Fever, sore throat, malaise, myalgias. Sandpaper rash that begins in the groin and axillae and extends to the trunk and extremities. Flushed face and circumoral pallor. Cervical LAD.
What are the complications of scarlet fever?	Post-strep glomerulonephritis, rheumatic fever
What is the treatment for scarlet fever?	Penicillin

What are the signs and symptoms of Varicella?	Multiple crops of lesions that develop from vesicles to crusts
What is a unique physical exam finding in the diagnosis of Varicella?	Dewdrops on a rose petal
Is the varicella vaccine live attenuated or inactivated?	Live attenuated
What is the treatment of choice for varicella?	Acyclovir
Aspirin use with varicella has been associated with which complication?	Reye's syndrome

ACUTE RHEUMATIC FEVER

Which heart valve is most commonly affected in rheumatic fever?	Mitral valve
Which titer is positive in acute rheumatic fever?	Antistreptolysin O titer is positive
Acute rheumatic fever occurs as a result of which preceding complication?	Complication of pharyngitis due to group A streptococcus
What is the criteria to diagnose acute rheumatic fever?	Jones criteria
What are the components of the Jones criteria?	J = joints affected (e.g., polyarthritis) O (looks like a heart) = carditis (e.g., pancarditis) N = nodules (subcutaneous) E = erythema marginatum S = sydenham chorea
What are the minor criteria?	Arthralgia, elevated ESR or CRP, fever, leukocytosis, or prolonged PR interval
Which medication is used as prophylaxis for acute rheumatic fever?	Benzathine penicillin G

CONGENITAL HEART DEFECTS

Where is the foramen ovale located?	Between right and left atria

ATRIAL SEPTAL DEFECT

What is an atrial septal defect?	An opening in the interatrial septum
What is the most common type of atrial septal defect?	Septum secundum
How do you describe the murmur heard on auscultation of atrial septal defect?	Soft, systolic ejection murmur at the pulmonic area (left second ICS) with a fixed, wide splitting of S2
What are the signs and symptoms of atrial septal defect?	Often asymptomatic. If severe, exercise intolerance, fatigue, palpitations
What is the gold standard for diagnosing atrial septal defect?	Transthoracic echocardiogram
What is the treatment for atrial septal defect?	Most resolve spontaneously. If severe, percutaneous closing or surgical patching

COARCTATION OF THE AORTA

What is coarctation of the aorta?	Narrowing of the aortic lumen at the distal arch and descending aorta
More common in males or females?	Two times more common in M > F
Which part of the aorta is typically affected by Coarctation of the Aorta? a) Ascending aorta b) Aortic arch c) Descending aorta d) Abdominal aorta	Answer: c) Descending aorta
What are the signs and symptoms?	May be asymptomatic. If severe, bilateral claudication, dyspnea on exertion, and syncope
What are the physical exam findings?	Upper extremity systolic hypertension with lower extremity hypotension +/- diminished lower extremity pulses such as femoral and dorsalis pedis

What murmur is heard upon auscultation?	Late systolic ejection murmur over left posterior hemithorax +/- continuous murmur that radiates to the posterior scapular area
What will you see on chest x-ray and why?	Posterior rib notching due to increased blood flow through the intercostal artery collateral circulation
What is the best diagnostic test for coarctation of the aorta?	Echo is confirmatory
What is the best initial treatment for coarctation of the aorta?	PEG1
What is the preferred treatment for Coarctation of the Aorta? a) Medication to manage blood pressure b) Surgical repair or balloon angioplasty c) Lifestyle modifications d) Monitoring without intervention	Answer: b) Surgical repair or balloon angioplasty

What is hypertrophic cardiomyopathy?	Hypertrophic Cardiomyopathy is a genetic heart condition characterized by abnormal thickening of the heart muscle, which can lead to various symptoms and complications.
What is the most common cause of sudden cardiac death in young athletes?	Hypertrophic cardiomyopathy
What are the signs and symptoms of hypertrophic cardiomyopathy?	Can be asymptomatic; or can manifest as chest pain, shortness of breath, palpitations, fatigue, dizziness, and fainting spells.
What does the murmur sound like in a patient diagnosed with hypertrophic cardiomyopathy?	Harsh mid-systolic crescendo-decrescendo murmur at left sternal border (radiates to apex and heard best at the 3rd/4th ICS.
How do you diagnose hypertrophic cardiomyopathy?	Transthoracic echocardiography with doppler
What is the treatment for hypertrophic cardiomyopathy?	Automated implantable cardioverter defibrillator. Pharm—first line: beta blockers (e.g., metoprolol). Second line: non-DHP CCBs (e.g., Verapamil)

What is the most common cause of acquired heart disease?	Kawasaki disease
What are the signs and symptoms of Kawasaki disease?	Lip/oral cavity changes (e.g., lip cracking, fissures, **strawberry tongue**), bilateral painless conjunctivitis, unilateral cervical LAD > 1.5cm, polymorphous exanthem, extremities are red and edematous
What are the criteria to diagnose Kawasaki disease?	Fever of at least 5 days AND at least 4 of the following: conjunctivitis, mucositis (e.g., strawberry tongue, fissured lips), polymorphous rash, extremity changes (e.g., erythema of palms and soles, edema of the hands/feet or desquamation of the hands/feet) and cervical LAD
What is the primary treatment for Kawasaki Disease? a) Antibiotics b) Antiviral medications c) Intravenous immunoglobulin (IVIG) and aspirin d) Steroid medications	Answer: c) Intravenous immunoglobulin (IVIG) and aspirin

Anatomically where is the ductus arteriosus located?	Between the pulmonary trunk and the aorta
Medication to close patent ductus arteriosus?	Indomethacin
Prostaglandin E on patent ductus arteriosus has what kind of effect?	Keeps the ductus arteriosus patent
What is heard on auscultation of ductus arteriosus on physical exam?	Continuous, harsh machine-like murmur at the 2nd intercostal space

SYNCOPE

What is syncope? **a) Sudden loss of consciousness due to insufficient blood flow to the brain** **b) Temporary muscle weakness and paralysis** **c) Abnormal heart rhythm causing chest pain** **d) Chronic inflammation of the lungs**	Answer: a) Sudden loss of consciousness due to insufficient blood flow to the brain
What are the common signs and symptoms of syncope?	Dizziness, lightheadedness, blurred vision, fainting, and loss of consciousness.
How is syncope diagnosed?	Thorough history, physical examination, and may include additional tests such as an electrocardiogram (ECG) and echocardiogram. Imaging tests like CT scan or MRI may be done if there is suspicion of structural abnormalities in the brain or heart. Lab tests are usually done to check for underlying conditions such as anemia, electrolyte imbalances, or cardiac enzymes if cardiac causes are suspected. Work-up also includes: check blood glucose, consider orthostatic hypotension, vasovagal, dehydration, CBC, CMP, BMP. Find underlying cause
What is the treatment for syncope?	Find the underlying cause. Non-pharmacological treatment options include avoiding triggers, maintaining proper hydration, wearing compression stockings, and lifestyle modifications. Medications may be prescribed depending on the underlying cause of syncope, such as beta-blockers for certain heart conditions or vasodilators for low blood pressure.

4 components of tetralogy of fallot?	Pulmonary stenosis Right ventricular hypertrophy Overriding aorta Ventricular septal defect
What does the murmur sound like on physical exam in the diagnosis of tetralogy of fallot?	Loud harsh systolic ejection murmur at the left sternal border
What is seen on chest radiograph in the workup of tetralogy of fallot?	Boot-shaped heart
What is the treatment for Tetralogy of Fallot?	Surgical intervention is the primary treatment, with the most common procedure being a total repair of the heart defects. Medications such as beta-blockers and diuretics may be used to manage symptoms and improve heart function. Examples may include propranolol, furosemide, and digoxin.

What is the most common congenital heart defect?	Ventricular septal defect
4-week-old baby with loud, harsh, holosystolic murmur at the LSB with palpable thrill, what is the diagnosis?	Ventricular septal defect, often associated with mitral regurgitation
What is the sound of the murmur heard on physical exam in the workup of ventricular septal defect?	Loud, harsh holosystolic murmur at the lower LSB, wide split S2
How do you diagnose ventricular septal defect?	CXR— cardiomegaly, pulmonary edema, increased pulmonary vasculature. EKG— left atrial and left ventricular hypertrophy. Confirmed by transthoracic echo (TTE)
What is the treatment for ventricular septal defect?	spontaneous resolution. If moderate-large, give diuretics, digoxin, potential surgical management

What is transposition of the great vessels (TGV)?	TGV is a congenital heart defect where the aorta and pulmonary artery are switched, resulting in a reversed blood flow.
What are the common signs and symptoms of transposition of the great vessels?	Cyanosis (bluish discoloration of the skin), difficulty breathing, poor feeding, and failure to thrive are common symptoms.
How do you diagnose transposition of the great vessels?	Diagnosis is typically made through a combination of physical examination, echocardiogram, and cardiac catheterization. Imaging tests such as echocardiography, cardiac MRI, and CT scan can provide detailed information about the heart's structure and blood flow.
Treatment for transposition of the great vessels?	Prostaglandin E1 (maintains a patent ductus arteriosus); or surgical intervention

APPENDICITIS

What is appendicitis?	Right lower quadrant pain due to acute inflammation of the appendix
What are the signs and symptoms of appendicitis?	Right lower quadrant pain, nausea, fever, anorexia
Which findings are seen on physical exam for appendicitis?	(+) McBurney, Rosving, Psoas, and obturator signs. Check for rebound tenderness and signs of peritoneal involvement
Which diagnostics are needed for the work up of appendicitis?	CBC (check for neutrophilia, leukocytosis with left shift, PMNs), BMP (look for elevated creatinine and electrolyte abnormalities), CRP, UA, imaging (e.g., u/s, CT scan with and without contrast)
What is the study of choice for appendicitis?	CT scan with IV contrast is the most accurate for diagnosing acute appendicitis
What is the treatment for appendicitis?	Get surgery consultation. Order 1 dose of Cefoxitin (Mefoxin)/Cefotetan (Cefotan) to prevent infection; 30-60min prior to incision; surgical appendectomy

COLIC

Colic is defined as: **A. Inflammation of the colon** **B. Persistent crying and fussiness in infants** **C. Abdominal pain in adults** **D. A bacterial infection in the gastrointestinal tract**	Answer: B Explanation: Colic refers to the persistent crying and fussiness in infants that lasts for several hours a day, usually occurring in the late afternoon or evening.
What is colic?	Severe paroxysmal crying (unexplained irritability and fussiness without a known cause/trigger)
What is the most common cause of colic in infants? **A. Gastroesophageal reflux disease (GERD)** **B. Milk allergy or intolerance** **C. Abdominal obstruction** **D. Infection of the gastrointestinal tract**	Answer: B Explanation: Milk allergy or intolerance is one of the most common causes of colic in infants. Cow's milk protein is often the culprit, and eliminating it from the diet can help alleviate symptoms.
How do you diagnose colic?	3 hours of crying per day for at least 3 days a week for a total of 3 weeks
What is the treatment for colic?	Patient education aimed at calming distressed parents and providing reassurance. Encourage dietary recommendations, regular diaper changes, decreasing stimulation, cradling, soothing, rocking, etc
Which of the following is an important measure for health maintenance in infants with colic? **A. Vaccination against gastrointestinal infections** **B. Regular follow-up with a pediatric gastroenterologist** **C. Adequate nutrition and hydration** **D. Daily administration of stool softeners**	Answer: C Explanation: Ensuring adequate nutrition and hydration is crucial for the overall health and well-being of infants with colic.

CONSTIPATION

How do you define constipation?	<3 bowel movement per week
What are the signs and symptoms of constipation?	Increased straining, passage of hard stools, nausea, abdominal pain, bloating, anorexia

What is the name of the criteria to diagnose constipation?	Rome IV
What is the treatment for constipation?	Non-pharm (e.g., fiber, increased fluids, bulk-forming laxatives). Pharm, if necessary (osmotic laxatives)

Which laboratory parameter is often used to assess dehydration? **A. Hemoglobin level** **B. Serum electrolyte levels** **C. C-reactive protein (CRP)** **D. Blood glucose level**	Answer: B Explanation: Serum electrolyte levels, such as sodium and potassium, are often assessed to evaluate the severity and type of dehydration.
How is dehydration defined?	Mild: No hemodynamic changes (about 5% body weight in infants and 3% in adolescents) Moderate: Tachycardia (about 10% body weight in infants and 5 to 6% in adolescents) Severe: Hypotension with impaired perfusion (about 15% body weight in infants and 7 to 9% in adolescents)
What is the first-line treatment for mild to moderate dehydration? **A. Intravenous (IV) fluids** **B. Oral rehydration solution** **C. Antibiotics** **D. Diuretics**	Answer: B Explanation: Oral rehydration solution is the first-line treatment for mild to moderate dehydration. It contains a balanced mixture of water, salts, and sugars to help replenish lost fluids.
In severe dehydration, intravenous fluids are often necessary. Which fluid is commonly used for intravenous rehydration? **A. Normal saline (0.9% sodium chloride)** **B. Dextrose solution** **C. Lactated Ringer's solution** **D. Sterile water**	Answer: A Explanation: Normal saline (0.9% sodium chloride) is commonly used for intravenous rehydration in severe dehydration. It helps restore electrolyte balance and fluid volume.
What is skin turgor?	Skin turgor refers to the elasticity and resilience of the skin. It is often assessed as a clinical indicator of hydration status. When the body is well-hydrated, the skin has good turgor and quickly returns to its normal position after being pinched or lifted. However, in cases of dehydration, the skin may have decreased turgor and may take longer to return to its original state. Poor skin turgor is often associated with decreased fluid intake or excessive fluid loss. Assessing skin turgor can help in evaluating the degree of dehydration in a patient.

What is duodenal atresia?	Complete occlusion or absence of duodenal lumen
The most common presentation of duodenal atresia in newborns is: **A. Bilious vomiting** **B. Non-bilious vomiting** **C. Severe diarrhea** **D. Abdominal distension**	Answer: A Explanation: The most common presentation of duodenal atresia in newborns is bilious vomiting, which is often described as "green vomit" due to the obstruction preventing the passage of bile into the intestine.

What are the signs and symptoms of duodenal atresia?

Bilious vomiting in the first two days of life (commonly after the first few hours of life), abdominal distention, and delayed meconium passage

What is the classic sign seen on x-ray for duodenal atresia?

Double bubble sign; air and fluid buildup separated by the pyloric sphincter (e.g., two "bubbles" seen on imaging–one in the stomach and one the duodenum)

What is double bubble sign?

Gas trapping in the stomach and the duodenum

Duodenal atresia is commonly associated with which genetic condition?
A. Down syndrome
B. Turner syndrome
C. Marfan syndrome
D. Fragile X syndrome

Answer: A
Explanation: Duodenal atresia is frequently associated with Down syndrome, with an estimated 30% to 40% of cases occurring in individuals with this genetic condition.

The treatment for duodenal atresia usually involves:
A. Antibiotic therapy
B. Surgical repair
C. Endoscopic dilation
D. Lifestyle modifications

Answer: B
Explanation: The standard treatment for duodenal atresia is surgical repair, which involves removing the obstruction and reestablishing the normal flow of food through the duodenum.

Encopresis is defined as:
A. Involuntary passage of stool in inappropriate places
B. Frequent urination during the day
C. Excessive sweating
D. Sudden loss of consciousness

Answer: A
Explanation: Encopresis refers to the involuntary or intentional passage of stool in inappropriate places, typically occurring in children beyond the age of expected toilet training.

What is the etiology for encopresis?

The primary etiology of encopresis is chronic constipation and fecal impaction, leading to involuntary stool leakage around the impacted feces.

The most common sign or symptom of encopresis is:
A. Frequent episodes of diarrhea
B. Abdominal pain and bloating
C. Blood in the stool
D. Soiling of underwear or clothing with stool

Answer: D
Explanation: The hallmark sign of encopresis is soiling of underwear or clothing with stool, often occurring due to involuntary leakage around the impacted feces.

What is the treatment for encopresis?

The primary non-pharmacological treatment for encopresis involves dietary modifications, such as a high-fiber diet and increased fluid intake, to promote regular bowel movements and prevent constipation. Pharmacological treatment options for encopresis often involve the use of stimulant laxatives and stool softeners to relieve constipation and facilitate regular bowel movements. Medications such as polyethylene glycol (PEG) are commonly used to treat constipation and encopresis by softening the stool and promoting regular bowel movements.

What is foreign body aspiration?

Foreign body swallowing refers to the accidental ingestion of objects that are not intended for ingestion, which can pose a risk of complications.

What imaging is ordered?

X-ray. Imaging studies such as X-rays may be used to detect the presence and location of foreign objects in the digestive tract.

| **What is the management?** | May involve endoscopic removal of the object to prevent complications. |
| **What are the complications of foreign body aspiration?** | Complications of foreign body swallowing can include gastrointestinal bleeding, especially if the object causes injury or irritation to the digestive tract. Most worrisome aspiration includes batteries or other toxic materials. |

GASTROENTERITIS

What is gastroenteritis?	Inflammation of the GI tract
What is the most common cause of gastroenteritis?	Viral gastroenteritis
Which type of pathogen is typically due to dairy products or deli-meats?	Listeria monocytogenes
Which pathogen causes bloody diarrhea and is due to poultry or unpasteurized milk	*Campylobacter* (e.g., *Campylobacter jejuni*)
Which gastroenteritis-causing pathogen is suspected in a patient with abdominal pain and bloody diarrhea with no fever?	Shiga toxin-producing E. Coli
What are the signs and symptoms of gastroenteritis?	Abdominal pain, NVD
Which labs are ordered in the workup of gastroenteritis?	CBC, CMP, UA, stool sample if necessary
T/F: Loperamide is recommended in the treatment of inflammatory diarrhea with a fever?	False. Avoid anti-motility drugs in a patient suspected of inflammatory diarrhea due to the risk of developing toxic megacolon
What is the treatment for gastroenteritis?	Supportive care, oral hydration, ondansetron (Zofran) for nausea

GASTROESOPHAGEAL REFLUX DISEASE

What is gastro-esophageal reflux disease (GERD)?	GERD is a chronic condition characterized by the backward flow of stomach acid into the esophagus, causing symptoms such as heartburn and regurgitation.
The primary cause of GERD is: **A. Genetic factors** **B. Excessive alcohol consumption** **C. Helicobacter pylori infection** **D. Dysfunction of the lower esophageal sphincter**	Answer: D Explanation: The primary cause of GERD is the dysfunction of the lower esophageal sphincter (LES), a muscular ring that normally prevents the backflow of stomach acid into the esophagus.
The diagnosis of GERD is typically made based on: **A. Blood tests** **B. Radiographic imaging of the esophagus** **C. Upper endoscopy (EGD)** **D. Stool analysis**	Answer: C Explanation: The diagnosis of GERD is typically made based on upper endoscopy (EGD), which allows direct visualization of the esophagus and identification of any abnormalities.
Complications of untreated GERD can include: **A. Pancreatitis** **B. Gallstones** **C. Barrett's esophagus** **D. Appendicitis**	Answer: C Explanation: Untreated GERD can lead to complications such as Barrett's esophagus, a condition where the lining of the esophagus undergoes cellular changes and increases the risk of esophageal cancer.
Non-pharmacological treatment options for GERD may include: **A. Dietary modifications** **B. Antibiotic therapy** **C. Radiation therapy** **D. Intravenous fluids**	Answer: A Explanation: Non-pharmacological treatment options for GERD include dietary modifications, such as avoiding trigger foods, maintaining a healthy weight, and elevating the head of the bed during sleep.
The first-line pharmacological treatment for GERD is usually:	Answer: A

A. Proton pump inhibitors (PPIs)
B. Antibiotics
C. Anticoagulants
D. Bronchodilators

Explanation: Proton pump inhibitors (PPIs) are the first-line pharmacological treatment for GERD. They reduce the production of stomach acid and help relieve symptoms. Can also use H2 receptor blockers

HEPATITIS

What is hepatitis?

Hepatitis refers to inflammation of the liver, which can be caused by viral infections, alcohol abuse, autoimmune diseases, or certain medications.

The most common cause of viral hepatitis worldwide is:
A. Hepatitis A virus (HAV)
B. Hepatitis B virus (HBV)
C. Hepatitis C virus (HCV)
D. Hepatitis D virus (HDV)

Answer: C
Explanation: Hepatitis C virus (HCV) is the most common cause of viral hepatitis worldwide, primarily transmitted through exposure to infected blood.

Hepatitis B virus (HBV) is primarily transmitted through:
A. Contaminated food and water
B. Sexual contact
C. Inhalation of respiratory droplets
D. Genetic inheritance

Answer: B
Explanation: Hepatitis B virus (HBV) is primarily transmitted through sexual contact, exposure to infected blood, or from an infected mother to her newborn.

The most specific diagnostic test for viral hepatitis is:
A. Liver biopsy
B. Complete blood count (CBC)
C. Hepatitis serology (blood tests)
D. Abdominal ultrasound

Answer: C
Explanation: Hepatitis serology, including specific blood tests for viral markers such as hepatitis B surface antigen (HBsAg) and hepatitis C antibody (anti-HCV), is the most specific diagnostic test for viral hepatitis.

Which type of hepatitis can lead to chronic liver disease, cirrhosis, and liver cancer?
A. Hepatitis A
B. Hepatitis B
C. Hepatitis C
D. Hepatitis D

Answer: C
Explanation: Hepatitis C (HCV) is the type of hepatitis that can lead to chronic liver disease, cirrhosis, and liver cancer if left untreated.

HIRSCHSPRUNG DISEASE

What is Hirschsprung disease?

Congenital loss of ganglion cells of the distal colon during development that leads to megacolon

Hirschsprung disease is associated with which genetic mutation?

Down syndrome (trisomy 21)

What are the signs and symptoms of Hirschsprung disease?

Failure to pass meconium, bilious vomiting, abdominal distention

What is the gold standard for diagnosing Hirschsprung disease?

Rectal biopsy

What is the treatment for Hirschsprung disease?

Surgical resection of affected bowel

INGUINAL HERNIA

Which type of inguinal hernia is the most common?

Indirect inguinal hernia

What are the boundaries of Hesselbach's triangle?

Inferior border: inguinal ligament
Medial border: rectus abdominis muscle
Superolateral border: inferior epigastric vessels

Which type of inguinal hernia passes through the inguinal canal?

Indirect inguinal hernia

Which type of inguinal hernia reaches the scrotum?

Indirect inguinal hernia

A direct inguinal hernia is medial or lateral to the inferior epigastric vessels?

Medial

| An indirect inguinal hernia is medial or lateral to the inferior epigastric vessels? | Lateral |

INTUSSUSCEPTION

What is Intussusception?	• Intestine folds into section next to it • Telescoping of the proximal segment into distal segment
Which type of stool is seen and considered pathognomonic for Intussusception?	Currant jelly stool
Which type of mass is felt on physical exam?	Sausage-like mass
Anatomically, where is Intussusception most common?	Ileocecal junction
What are the signs and symptoms of Intussusception?	Acute onset cyclical colicky abdominal pain, legs drawn up to chest with asymptomatic episodes in between
What is the classic triad for Intussusception?	Abdominal pain, palpable sausage-like mass palpated on RUQ, and currant jelly stool
If Intussusception, which test should be ordered?	Contrast enema
What is the best test to confirm Intussusception?	Contrast enema
Which sign is seen on abdominal u/s?	Target sign; the invaginated portion of bowel appears as rings on a target on u/s
What is the treatment of choice?	Air enema

JAUNDICE

What is jaundice?	Jaundice is characterized by the yellowing of the skin and eyes due to an excess of bilirubin, a yellow pigment produced during the breakdown of red blood cells.
The most common cause of jaundice is: A. Liver cirrhosis B. Gallstones C. Hepatitis A infection D. Excessive alcohol consumption	Answer: A Explanation: Liver cirrhosis is the most common cause of jaundice, where the liver becomes scarred and unable to function properly.
Elevated levels of which substance in the blood lead to jaundice? A. Uric acid B. Hemoglobin C. Bilirubin D. Cholesterol	Answer: C Explanation: Jaundice occurs due to the accumulation of bilirubin in the bloodstream, which can result from liver disease or obstruction of the bile ducts.
Treatment of jaundice depends on the underlying cause and may include: A. Surgery to remove the gallbladder B. Medications to dissolve gallstones C. Antiviral therapy for viral hepatitis D. All of the above	Answer: D Explanation: Treatment of jaundice depends on the underlying cause. It may include surgery to remove the gallbladder in the case of gallstones, medications to dissolve gallstones, and antiviral therapy for viral hepatitis.

LACTOSE INTOLERANCE

What is lactose intolerance?	Lactose intolerance is the inability to digest lactose, a sugar found in milk and dairy products, due to insufficient production of lactase, the enzyme responsible for breaking down lactose.
What are common symptoms of lactose intolerance?	Abdominal pain and bloating, diarrhea, and constipation are frequently reported symptoms.
What is the definitive diagnosis for lactose intolerance?	Lactose hydrogen breath test

What is the treatment for lactose intolerance?	Avoidance of dairy; +/- lactase supplements

What is the primary source of niacin?	Fish and seafood are primary dietary sources of niacin. Other sources include meat, poultry, legumes, and fortified cereals.
What is Pellagra?	Pellagra, a manifestation of niacin deficiency, is characterized by the "3 Ds": dermatitis (dry, scaly skin), diarrhea, and dementia. Other symptoms may include a swollen tongue, fatigue, and weakness.
Niacin deficiency can be prevented or treated by: **A. Increasing sun exposure** **B. Consuming niacin-rich foods** **C. Taking niacin supplements** **D. All of the above**	Answer: D Explanation: Niacin deficiency can be prevented or treated by increasing intake of niacin-rich foods, such as fish and seafood, and by taking niacin supplements under medical supervision.
Severe niacin deficiency can lead to: **A. Scurvy** **B. Rickets** **C. Pellagra** **D. Beriberi**	Answer: C Explanation: Severe niacin deficiency can lead to pellagra, a condition characterized by the "3 Ds" (dermatitis, diarrhea, and dementia).

What is pyloric stenosis?	Hypertrophy and hyperplasia of the pyloric sphincter
What are the signs and symptoms of pyloric sphincter?	Regurgitation, non-bilious, projectile vomiting after feeding
Which shaped mass may be palpated on physical exam?	Olive-shaped mass palpated on RUQ
What results are seen on laboratory tests?	Hypochloremic, hypokalemic metabolic alkalosis
What is the best initial imaging?	Abdominal u/s
What is the treatment for pyloric stenosis?	Conservative management–correct electrolyte imbalances, IV rehydration. If severe–pyloromyotomy

An umbilical hernia is characterized by: **A. Protrusion of abdominal organs through the umbilical ring** **B. Protrusion of abdominal organs through the inguinal canal** **C. Protrusion of abdominal organs through the diaphragm** **D. Protrusion of abdominal organs through the umbilical vessels**	Answer: A Explanation: An umbilical hernia is characterized by the protrusion of abdominal organs (such as intestines) through the umbilical ring in the abdominal wall.
What are the risk factors for umbilical hernia?	Risk factors for developing an umbilical hernia include obesity, pregnancy (due to increased abdominal pressure), and chronic coughing or straining.
The main symptom of an umbilical hernia is: **A. Pain and discomfort at the hernia site** **B. Nausea and vomiting** **C. Redness and swelling around the umbilicus** **D. Visible bulge or protrusion at the umbilicus**	Answer: D Explanation: The main symptom of an umbilical hernia is a visible bulge or protrusion at the umbilicus, which becomes more noticeable during activities that increase intra-abdominal pressure (such as crying or straining).

What are the fat-soluble vitamins?	Vitamin ADEK

What are the sources of vitamin A? — Liver, kidney, eggs, butter, leafy vegetables

What is the function of vitamin A? — Vision (retinal pigments), immune health

NIACIN (B3) DEFICIENCY

What are sources of vitamin B3? — Meat (e.g., liver), seeds, legumes

VITAMIN C DEFICIENCY

What are the sources of vitamin C? — Fruits (e.g., citrus, strawberries), vegetables (e.g., cabbage, spinach)

What are the signs and symptoms of vitamin C deficiency? — Hyperkeratosis, hemorrhage (e.g., gums, skin, joints), anemia, and glossitis

Vitamin C deficiency causes which disease? — Scurvy

VITAMIN D DEFICIENCY

What are the risk factors for vitamin D deficiency? — Inadequate sun exposure, absence of fortified dairy, exclusive breastfeeding in infants

A vitamin D deficiency may cause which disease? — Rickets

What are the signs and symptoms of Rickets? — Bowed legs, fractures, symptoms of hypocalcemia (e.g., tetany, paresthesias)

VOLVULUS

What is volvulus? — Twisting of a loop of bowel on its mesentery that can lead to obstruction

Which anatomical location is most commonly affected in children with volvulus? — Midgut volvulus

What are the signs and symptoms of volvulus? — Bilious vomiting, hemodynamic instability, and abdominal distention

What is seen on CT scan of the abdomen and pelvis? — Whirlpool sign (suggests midgut volvulus)

What is the gold standard for the diagnosis of volvulus? — Upper GI series

ANTICIPATORY GUIDANCE

The goal of anticipatory guidance is to:
A. Prevent future health problems and promote healthy child development
B. Diagnose and treat existing health conditions in children
C. Provide immediate solutions to parental concerns and questions
D. Educate parents on common childhood illnesses

Answer: A
Explanation: The goal of anticipatory guidance is to prevent future health problems and promote healthy child development by providing parents with information and strategies to support their child's physical, emotional, and social well-being.

Which of the following is a typical developmental milestone for a 6-month-old infant?
A. Crawling
B. Walking independently
C. Speaking in sentences
D. Feeding with a spoon

Answer: A
Explanation: Crawling is a typical developmental milestone for a 6-month-old infant. Walking independently usually occurs around 12-15 months, speaking in sentences around 2 years, and feeding with a spoon around 9-12 months.

Anticipatory guidance topics may include:
A. Nutrition and healthy eating habits
B. Safety and injury prevention
C. Developmental milestones
D. All of the above

Answer: D
Explanation: Anticipatory guidance topics commonly include nutrition and healthy eating habits, safety and injury prevention, developmental milestones, behavior management, and other aspects of child care and development.

Which of the following is an example of anticipatory guidance for safety?
A. Discussing the importance of using car seats and seat belts correctly
B. Providing information on child development milestones
C. Advising on age-appropriate toys and activities
D. Explaining the benefits of immunizations

Answer: A
Explanation: Discussing the importance of using car seats and seat belts correctly is an example of anticipatory guidance for safety, as it addresses a potential hazard and provides guidance on how to protect the child from hazards.

Which of the following may be a sign of child abuse?
A. Frequent falls or accidents
B. Fear of going to school
C. Eager participation in age-appropriate activities
D. Consistent weight gain and growth

Answer: B
Explanation: Fear of going to school may be a sign of child abuse, indicating potential emotional or physical mistreatment.

The leading cause of unintentional injury-related deaths in children aged 1-4 years is:
A. Drowning
B. Burns
C. Poisoning
D. Motor vehicle accidents

Answer: A
Explanation: Drowning is the leading cause of unintentional injury-related deaths in children aged 1-4 years. It is important to ensure appropriate water safety measures and supervision to prevent drowning incidents.

How should poisonings in children be managed?
A. Inducing vomiting immediately
B. Offering plenty of fluids to dilute the toxin
C. Contacting a poison control center or seeking medical attention
D. Administering over-the-counter pain relievers

Answer: C
Explanation: Poisonings in children should be managed by contacting a poison control center or seeking immediate medical attention. Inducing vomiting or administering any treatments should only be done under professional guidance.

What is the recommended approach for addressing potential signs of abuse in children?
A. Ignore the signs unless they persist for an extended period
B. Confront the caregiver without involving authorities
C. Report suspicions to the appropriate child protective services
D. Document the signs but refrain from taking further action

Answer: C
Explanation: The recommended approach for addressing potential signs of abuse in children is to report suspicions to the appropriate child protective services, allowing professionals to investigate and ensure the child's safety.

DOWN SYNDROME

What is Down syndrome?

Down syndrome is a genetic disorder caused by the presence of an extra copy of chromosome 21. It is also known as Trisomy 21.

What are the risks for developing Down syndrome?

The main risk factor for Down syndrome is maternal age, with an increased likelihood in pregnancies of women over 35 years old. However, it can occur in pregnancies of women of any age.

What are the signs and symptoms of Down syndrome?

Common signs and symptoms of Down syndrome include intellectual disability, distinct facial features (such as almond-shaped eyes and a flat nasal bridge), poor muscle tone, developmental delays, and an increased risk of certain health conditions.

How is Down syndrome diagnosed?

Down syndrome can be diagnosed prenatally through tests such as amniocentesis or chorionic villus sampling (CVS), which analyze fetal cells for chromosomal abnormalities. It can also be diagnosed after birth based on physical characteristics and confirmed through genetic testing.

What is the treatment for Down syndrome?

There is no cure for Down syndrome, but early intervention programs can help address developmental delays and provide support for individuals with Down syndrome and their families. Treatment focuses on managing associated health conditions, promoting education and social inclusion, and providing supportive care.

FEBRILE SEIZURE

What are febrile seizures?

Febrile seizures are convulsions that occur in young children, usually between the ages of 6 months and 5 years, as a result of a sudden spike in body temperature, often due to an underlying infection.

What are the risk factors for developing febrile seizures?

The main risk factors for febrile seizures include a family history of febrile seizures, younger age, and a lower fever threshold.

What are the signs and symptoms of febrile seizures?

Febrile seizures are typically generalized and characterized by sudden convulsions, loss of consciousness, and uncontrolled shaking or jerking of the limbs. They are often brief and do not cause long-term neurological damage.

A 9-month-old infant presents with a brief seizure lasting for about 1 minute. The parents report that the child had a fever for the past 2 days, and the temperature was recorded as 38.5°C (101.3°F). The

Answer: C) Observation and reassurance
Explanation: In a young child with a simple febrile seizure and no concerning features, the most appropriate management is observation and

child appears well and has no other concerning symptoms. What is the most appropriate management?
A) Admission to the hospital for further evaluation
B) Lumbar puncture to rule out meningitis
C) Observation and reassurance
D) Initiation of antiepileptic medication

reassurance. Hospital admission and invasive procedures like lumbar puncture are generally not indicated.

IMMUNIZATION GUIDELINES

A 6-month-old infant presents to the clinic for a routine check-up. According to the immunization schedule, which vaccines should the infant receive at this visit?
A) Hepatitis B, Rotavirus, Diphtheria-tetanus-acellular pertussis (DTaP), Haemophilus influenzae type b (Hib)
B) Inactivated polio vaccine (IPV), Pneumococcal conjugate vaccine (PCV), Influenza
C) Measles-mumps-rubella (MMR), Varicella, Hepatitis A
D) Tetanus-diphtheria-acellular pertussis (Tdap), Human papillomavirus (HPV)

Answer: A) Hepatitis B, Rotavirus, Diphtheria-tetanus-acellular pertussis (DTaP), Haemophilus influenzae type b (Hib)

Explanation: At 6 months of age, the recommended vaccines include Hepatitis B, Rotavirus, DTaP, and Hib vaccines.

Which of the following vaccines is typically given at birth?
A) Pneumococcal conjugate vaccine (PCV)
B) Hepatitis B vaccine
C) Influenza vaccine
D) Meningococcal conjugate vaccine (MCV)

Answer: B) Hepatitis B vaccine

Explanation: The Hepatitis B vaccine is typically administered to newborns within the first 24 hours of life.

Which of the following is an example of active immunity?
A) Receiving preformed antibodies through immunoglobulin administration
B) Receiving a vaccine to stimulate an immune response
C) Transferring antibodies from a pregnant mother to her fetus
D) Developing immunity after recovering from an illness

Answer: B) Receiving a vaccine to stimulate an immune response

Explanation: Active immunity is achieved when the immune system is stimulated to produce its own immune response, such as through vaccination.

Which of the following vaccines is typically administered to adolescents to prevent cervical cancer?
A) Hepatitis B vaccine
B) Influenza vaccine
C) Human papillomavirus (HPV) vaccine
D) Meningococcal conjugate vaccine (MCV)

Answer: C) Human papillomavirus (HPV)

Explanation: the HPV vaccine is recommended for adolescents against certain strains of HPV which can cause cervical cancer

MENINGITIS

A 21-year-old college student presents to the emergency department with sudden onset of severe headache, high fever, neck stiffness, and sensitivity to light. The patient appears lethargic. Which of the following is the most appropriate initial step in management?
A) Lumbar puncture for cerebrospinal fluid (CSF) analysis

Answer: B) Administration of broad-spectrum antibiotics

Explanation: Based on the patient's clinical presentation of severe headache, high fever, neck stiffness, and altered mental status, there is a high suspicion for bacterial meningitis. Immediate

B) Administration of broad-spectrum antibiotics
C) Brain MRI
D) Blood culture

Which of the following organisms is the most common cause of bacterial meningitis in infants aged 1-3 months?
A) Neisseria meningitidis
B) Streptococcus pneumoniae
C) Group B Streptococcus
D) Haemophilus influenzae type b

Which of the following diagnostic tests is the gold standard for diagnosing meningitis?
A) Blood culture
B) Lumbar puncture for CSF analysis
C) CT scan of the head
D) Polymerase chain reaction (PCR) testing

Which of the following vaccines is included in routine childhood immunizations to prevent meningitis caused by Haemophilus influenzae type b?
A) Measles-mumps-rubella (MMR) vaccine
B) Varicella vaccine
C) Pneumococcal conjugate vaccine (PCV)
D) Hib vaccine

administration of broad-spectrum antibiotics is crucial to cover the most common pathogens.

Answer: C) Group B Streptococcus

Explanation: Group B Streptococcus is the most common cause of bacterial meningitis in infants aged 1-3 months. Streptococcus pneumoniae is the most common cause in older children and adults.

Answer: B) Lumbar puncture for CSF analysis

Explanation: Lumbar puncture with CSF analysis, including cell count, glucose, protein levels, and gram stain/culture, is the gold standard for diagnosing meningitis and determining the causative organism.

Answer: D) Hib vaccine

Explanation: The Hib vaccine is part of routine childhood immunizations and helps prevent invasive disease caused by Haemophilus influenzae type b, including meningitis.

NORMAL GROWTH AND DEVELOPMENT

A 4-month-old infant is brought to the pediatrician for a routine check-up. The infant is able to lift their head while lying on their stomach, smiles in response to social interactions, and reaches for objects with both hands. Which of the following developmental milestones is the infant most likely demonstrating?
A) Rolling over
B) Sitting without support
C) Crawling
D) Grasping objects

Answer: D) Grasping objects

Explanation: By 4 months of age, infants typically exhibit the ability to lift their head, smile in response to social interactions, and reach for objects with both hands. Grasping objects is an important milestone at this age.

Which of the following is a common gross motor milestone achieved by a 12-month-old infant?
A) Walking independently
B) Jumping with both feet
C) Climbing stairs
D) Riding a tricycle

Answer: A) Walking independently

Explanation: Walking independently is a typical gross motor milestone achieved by a 12-month-old infant. Climbing stairs typically occurs around 18 months, jumping with both feet around 2-3 years, and riding a tricycle around 3 years.

During which stage of development do children typically experience a rapid growth in language skills, start using two-word phrases, and show an increased curiosity about their environment?
A) Infancy (0-12 months)
B) Toddlerhood (1-3 years)
C) Preschool age (3-5 years)
D) School age (6-12 years)

Answer: B) Toddlerhood (1-3 years)

Explanation: Toddlerhood is characterized by a rapid growth in language skills, including the use of two-word phrases (around 18-24 months), and increased curiosity about the environment.

Which vaccine is routinely recommended for all adolescents at the age of 11-12 years?
A) Influenza

Answer: C) Tdap

B) Meningococcal conjugate
C) Tdap
D) Hepatitis A

A 9-year-old child is experiencing increased peer interactions and friendships. This reflects the developmental milestone known as:
A) Egocentrism.
B) Identity vs. role confusion.
C) Industry vs. inferiority.
D) Social competence.

A 12-year-old girl is brought in for a check-up. The parents report that she has recently experienced a growth spurt and has started developing breast buds. What is the typical age range for the onset of breast development in girls?
A) 6-8 years
B) 8-10 years
C) 10-12 years
D) 12-14 years

A 15-year-old boy is seen in the clinic. He is concerned about his short stature compared to his peers. His parents report a family history of delayed growth. What condition should be considered in this teenager?
A) Turner syndrome
B) Down syndrome
C) Klinefelter syndrome
D) Constitutional growth delay

Explanation: The Tdap vaccine, which provides protection against tetanus, diphtheria, and pertussis, is routinely recommended for all adolescents at the age of 11-12 years.

Answer: D) Social competence.

Explanation: Social competence, characterized by increased peer interactions, friendships, and cooperation, is a key developmental milestone during middle childhood (around 6-12 years of age).

Answer: C) 10-12 years

Explanation: The typical age range for the onset of breast development (thelarche) in girls is between 10 and 12 years. This marks the beginning of puberty.

Answer: D) Constitutional growth delay

Explanation: Constitutional growth delay is a common cause of delayed growth in adolescents. It is usually a familial trait and not associated with any underlying medical conditions. These teenagers experience delayed puberty and catch up in growth later during adolescence. Turner syndrome, Down syndrome, and Klinefelter syndrome typically present with additional features beyond short stature.

SEIZURE DISORDERS

What is a seizure?

A seizure is a sudden, abnormal electrical discharge in the brain that results in a temporary disruption of brain function.

What is epilepsy?

Epilepsy is a chronic neurological disorder characterized by recurrent, unprovoked seizures.

What are the two main categories of seizures?

The two main categories of seizures are focal (partial) seizures and generalized seizures.

What are focal (partial) seizures?

Focal seizures originate in a specific area of the brain and may or may not spread to other parts. They can be classified as focal aware seizures or focal impaired awareness seizures.

What are generalized seizures?

Generalized seizures involve both cerebral hemispheres from the onset and typically result in loss of consciousness. They can be further classified into several subtypes, including absence seizures, tonic-clonic seizures, and myoclonic seizures.

What are some common causes of seizures?

Common causes of seizures include epilepsy, brain tumors, head injuries, stroke, infections (such as meningitis or encephalitis), genetic disorders, and metabolic imbalances.

What are some signs and symptoms of a seizure?	Signs and symptoms of a seizure can vary depending on the type but may include convulsions, loss of consciousness, abnormal movements or behavior, confusion, staring spells, and temporary loss of memory.
What are the treatment options for seizure disorders?	Treatment options for seizure disorders include antiepileptic medications (such as phenytoin, carbamazepine, or valproic acid), ketogenic diet, vagus nerve stimulation, and in some cases, surgical intervention.
What is status epilepticus?	Status epilepticus is a medical emergency characterized by prolonged seizures or a series of seizures without full recovery between them. It requires immediate medical intervention to prevent complications and brain damage.

TEETHING

At what age does teething typically occur?	Teething typically begins around 6 months of age, but it can vary between 4 and 10 months.
What are the signs and symptoms of teething?	Signs and symptoms of teething may include drooling, swollen or sensitive gums, irritability, chewing on objects, decreased appetite, disrupted sleep, and sometimes mild fever.
Which teeth are usually the first to appear during teething?	The lower central incisors (bottom front teeth) are usually the first to appear during teething.
What are some strategies to relieve teething discomfort?	Strategies to relieve teething discomfort include giving the baby a chilled teething ring or clean, cold washcloth to chew on, gently massaging the gums, providing appropriate pain relief medications (such as acetaminophen) as recommended by a healthcare provider, and providing comfort and reassurance to the baby.
When should the baby start seeing a dentist for routine dental care?	The American Academy of Pediatrics recommends that children see a dentist by their first birthday or within six months after the first tooth erupts, whichever comes first.

TURNER SYNDROME

What is the karyotype seen in tuner syndrome?	45, XO karyotype (e.g., offspring does not receive X or Y from father)
What is the most common cause of turner syndrome?	Primary amenorrhea
What are the signs and symptoms of turner syndrome?	Short and stocky stature, shield chest (e.g., broad and flat), widely spaced nipples, webbed neck, high-arched palate, short 4th metacarpal, low-set hairline, cubitus valgus, genu valgum, and scant pubic hair
Which labs should be ordered in the workup for turner syndrome?	Karyotype analysis, fertility testing, TSH, free T4 or total T4, ↓ estrogen, ↓ androgens, ↑ FSH, ↑ LH, anti-Mullerian hormone (AMH), renal u/s
What are the complications of turner syndrome?	Coarctation of the aorta, aortic dissection, hypertension, horseshoe kidney, Hashimoto thyroiditis, T2DM
What is the treatment for turner syndrome?	Cardiology consultation (e.g., EKG, echo, cardiac MRI), treat HTN (e.g., beta blockers or ACE inhibitors), estrogen and progesterone substitution,

growth hormone therapy, treat lymphedema, health maintenance (e.g., monitor BP, audiological exams, eye exams, monitor growth curves, annual physical exams)

ANXIETY DISORDERS
GENERALIZED ANXIETY DISORDER (GAD)

What is Generalized Anxiety Disorder (GAD)?
Generalized Anxiety Disorder is a chronic condition characterized by excessive, uncontrollable worry and anxiety about everyday events and activities.

What are the signs and symptoms of GAD?
Common signs and symptoms include persistent worry, restlessness, irritability, sleep disturbances, difficulty concentrating, and physical symptoms such as muscle tension and fatigue.

How is GAD diagnosed?
GAD is diagnosed based on the presence of excessive worrying and anxiety that persists for at least six months, along with associated symptoms that significantly impact daily life.

What are some non-pharmacological treatments for GAD?
Non-pharmacological treatments for GAD include cognitive-behavioral therapy (CBT), relaxation techniques, stress management, and lifestyle modifications such as regular exercise and healthy sleep habits.

What are the commonly used pharmacological treatments for GAD?
Selective serotonin reuptake inhibitors (SSRIs) and selective norepinephrine reuptake inhibitors (SNRIs) are commonly prescribed as first-line pharmacotherapy for GAD. Benzodiazepines may be used for short-term relief of symptoms.

OTHER ANXIETY DISORDERS

Which of the following is a defining characteristic of anxiety disorders?
A) Intrusive thoughts
B) Panic attacks
C) Specific phobias
D) Hyperactivity

Explanation: B) Panic attacks. While intrusive thoughts and specific phobias are related to anxiety disorders, panic attacks are a defining characteristic of anxiety disorders as a whole.

What is the most common phobic disorder?
A) Agoraphobia
B) Social anxiety disorder
C) Specific phobia
D) Panic disorder

Explanation: C) Specific phobia. Specific phobia is the most common phobic disorder, characterized by an intense and irrational fear of a specific object or situation.

Which of the following is a common risk factor for developing post-traumatic stress disorder (PTSD)?
A) Female gender
B) Advanced age
C) Family history of anxiety disorders
D) Previous traumatic event

Explanation: D) Previous traumatic event. Experiencing a previous traumatic event is a significant risk factor for developing PTSD.

What is the primary diagnostic criteria for adjustment disorders?
A) Excessive worrying about specific objects or situations
B) Presence of intrusive thoughts and flashbacks
C) Development of emotional or behavioral symptoms within three months of a stressor

Explanation: C) Development of emotional or behavioral symptoms within three months of a stressor. The primary diagnostic criteria for adjustment disorders is the development of emotional or behavioral symptoms in response to an identifiable stressor within three months.

D) Recurrent panic attacks and fear of future attacks

Which of the following laboratory tests is not typically indicated for the diagnosis of anxiety disorders, phobic disorders, PTSD, or adjustment disorders?
A) Complete blood count (CBC)
B) Thyroid function tests
C) Neuroimaging (e.g., MRI)
D) Urine drug screen

Explanation: C) Neuroimaging (e.g., MRI). Routine neuroimaging is not typically indicated for the diagnosis of anxiety disorders, phobic disorders, PTSD, or adjustment disorders. It may be ordered if there are specific indications or concerns of underlying neurological conditions.

What is a key component in the diagnosis of specific phobias?
A) Physical symptoms such as panic attacks
B) Persistent avoidance of the feared object or situation
C) History of traumatic events
D) Presence of intrusive thoughts

Explanation: B) Persistent avoidance of the feared object or situation. A key component in the diagnosis of specific phobias is the persistent avoidance of the feared object or situation due to intense fear or anxiety.

What is the first-line treatment for post-traumatic stress disorder (PTSD)?
A) Selective serotonin reuptake inhibitors (SSRIs)
B) Benzodiazepines
C) Antipsychotics
D) Tricyclic antidepressants (TCAs)

Explanation: A) Selective serotonin reuptake inhibitors (SSRIs). SSRIs are considered the first-line treatment for PTSD due to their efficacy in reducing symptoms and managing associated conditions like depression and anxiety.

Which of the following is an important aspect of patient education for individuals with phobic disorders?
A) Encouraging avoidance of all feared objects or situations
B) Gradual exposure to the feared object or situation
C) Limiting social interactions to minimize anxiety triggers
D) Restricting caffeine consumption

Explanation: B) Gradual exposure to the feared object or situation. Patient education for phobic disorders emphasizes gradual exposure therapy, where individuals are gradually exposed to the feared object or situation to reduce anxiety over time.

ATTENTION-DEFICIT/HYPERACTIVITY DISORDER (ADHD)

Diagnosis requires symptoms for at least how many months?	6 months
How many different settings are required to make the diagnosis?	At least two different settings (e.g., home, school, after-school programs, sports, etc)
Name on psychostimulant that is used in the treatment of ADHD?	Methylphenidate
What is the mechanism of methylphenidate?	Norepinephrine and dopamine reuptake inhibitor

AUTISM SPECTRUM DISORDER

Which of the following is a defining characteristic of Autism Spectrum Disorders (ASD)?
A) Hyperactivity and impulsivity
B) Excessive social interactions
C) Restricted and repetitive behaviors
D) Intense fear of social situations

Explanation: C) Restricted and repetitive behaviors. A key characteristic of ASD is the presence of restricted and repetitive behaviors, interests, or activities.

Which of the following is a recognized risk factor for Autism Spectrum Disorders (ASD)?
A) Maternal age
B) Breastfeeding

Explanation: A) Maternal age. Advanced maternal age is recognized as a risk factor for ASD, with a higher incidence observed in children born to older mothers.

C) Parental education level
D) Blood type
What is an important aspect of treatment for individuals with Autism Spectrum Disorder (ASD)?
A) Medication with stimulant drugs
B) Psychotherapy focusing on self-esteem
C) Applied Behavior Analysis (ABA) therapy
D) Hypnotherapy

Explanation: C) Applied Behavior Analysis (ABA) therapy. A key aspect of treatment for individuals with ASD is the use of evidence-based interventions such as Applied Behavior Analysis (ABA) therapy, which focuses on improving social skills and reducing problem behaviors.

CHILD ABUSE AND NEGLECT

What is the most common form of child maltreatment?
A) Physical abuse
B) Emotional abuse
C) Neglect
D) Sexual abuse

Explanation: C) Neglect. Neglect is the most common form of child maltreatment and refers to the failure to provide for a child's basic needs, including food, shelter, supervision, and medical care.

Which of the following is a risk factor for child abuse and neglect?
A) Adequate social support system
B) Stable socioeconomic status
C) History of substance abuse in the family
D) Parental history of high educational attainment

Explanation: C) History of substance abuse in the family. A history of substance abuse in the family is a recognized risk factor for child abuse and neglect, as it can contribute to impaired parenting abilities and compromised family dynamics.

What is a key aspect of treatment for child abuse and neglect?
A) Medication with psychotropic drugs
B) Individual therapy for the child
C) Family counseling and support services
D) Removal of the child from the home

Explanation: C) Family counseling and support services. Treatment for child abuse and neglect often involves comprehensive interventions, including family counseling and support services aimed at addressing the underlying issues, promoting healthy parenting skills, and ensuring the child's safety.

Sarah, a 6-year-old girl, is brought to the pediatrician by her teacher who notices multiple unexplained bruises on her arms and legs during a routine class activity. Sarah appears anxious and avoids making eye contact. Upon further questioning, the teacher learns that Sarah often arrives at school hungry and unkempt, and she seems withdrawn compared to her peers. Based on the patient's presentation, what is the most likely form of child maltreatment?
A) Physical abuse
B) Emotional abuse
C) Neglect
D) Sexual abuse

Answer: A) Physical abuse.

Explanation: The presence of unexplained bruises and the teacher's observation of Sarah's withdrawal and anxious behavior suggest physical abuse as the most likely form of maltreatment.

DEPRESSIVE DISORDERS

What is the primary characteristic of Major Depressive Disorder (MDD)?
A) Excessive happiness and euphoria
B) Rapid mood swings between highs and lows
C) Prolonged feelings of sadness and despair
D) Intense fear of social situations

Explanation: C) Prolonged feelings of sadness and despair. The primary characteristic of MDD is the presence of a depressed mood or loss of interest in almost all activities, persisting for at least two weeks.

What is believed to be a major contributing factor to the development of Major Depressive Disorder (MDD)?
A) Personal weakness or character flaws
B) Neurotransmitter imbalance in the brain

Explanation: B) Neurotransmitter imbalance in the brain. While the exact cause of MDD is unknown, it is believed to involve a combination of genetic, environmental, and neurochemical factors, including

C) Chronic pain conditions
D) Excessive social media use

Which of the following is a common symptom of Major Depressive Disorder (MDD)?
A) Hypomania
B) Delusions
C) Anhedonia
D) Hallucinations

imbalances in neurotransmitters such as serotonin, norepinephrine, and dopamine.

Answer: C) Anhedonia

Explanation: Anhedonia, the diminished ability to experience pleasure or interest in activities, is a common symptom of Major Depressive Disorder (MDD). Individuals with MDD often lose interest in activities they once enjoyed, and this lack of pleasure can contribute to feelings of emptiness and despair.

What is the first-line pharmacological treatment for Major Depressive Disorder (MDD)?
A) Selective serotonin reuptake inhibitors (SSRIs)
B) Benzodiazepines
C) Tricyclic antidepressants (TCAs)
D) Antipsychotics

Answer: A) Selective serotonin reuptake inhibitors (SSRIs)

Explanation: Selective serotonin reuptake inhibitors (SSRIs) are considered the first-line pharmacological treatment for Major Depressive Disorder (MDD). SSRIs work by increasing the availability of serotonin in the brain, which helps regulate mood. They have been shown to be effective in reducing depressive symptoms and are generally well-tolerated.

Which of the following is an appropriate initial step in the evaluation of a patient suspected to have MDD?
A) Ordering brain imaging (CT or MRI)
B) Assessing the patient's social support system
C) Conducting genetic testing for depressive disorders
D) Performing a complete blood count (CBC)

Answer: B) Assessing the patient's social support system

Explanation: When evaluating a patient suspected to have MDD, it is important to assess the patient's social support system. The presence or absence of a support system can influence the prognosis and guide treatment decisions. Ordering brain imaging, genetic testing, or a complete blood count is generally not indicated as initial steps in the evaluation of MDD unless there are specific clinical indications.

Which of the following psychotherapies has been shown to be effective in the treatment of MDD?
A) Psychodynamic therapy
B) Thought stopping technique
C) Cognitive-Behavioral Therapy (CBT)
D) Electroconvulsive therapy (ECT)

Answer: C) Cognitive-Behavioral Therapy (CBT)

Explanation: Cognitive-Behavioral Therapy (CBT) has been shown to be effective in the treatment of MDD. CBT focuses on identifying and modifying negative thought patterns and behaviors associated with depression. Psychodynamic therapy may be used in certain cases, but CBT has the strongest evidence base. Thought stopping technique is a technique used within therapy but not a standalone psychotherapy. Electroconvulsive therapy (ECT) is a treatment option for severe and treatment-resistant depression.

Which of the following is a second-line pharmacological treatment for MDD, often used in cases of treatment resistance?
A) Bupropion
B) Sertraline
C) Venlafaxine
D) Escitalopram

Answer: C) Venlafaxine

Explanation: Venlafaxine is considered a second-line pharmacological treatment for MDD, particularly in cases of treatment resistance. It is a serotonin-norepinephrine reuptake inhibitor (SNRI) and is prescribed at higher doses compared to selective serotonin reuptake inhibitors (SSRIs).

Which of the following is an example of a monoamine oxidase inhibitor (MAOI) used in the treatment of refractory depression?
A) Fluoxetine
B) Escitalopram

Answer: C) Tranylcypromine

Explanation: Tranylcypromine is an example of a monoamine oxidase inhibitor (MAOI) used in the treatment of refractory depression. MAOIs are

C) Tranylcypromine
D) Sertraline

What is the recommended dosage range for fluoxetine, a commonly prescribed SSRI for MDD?
A) 20-40 mg/day
B) 50-100 mg/day
C) 150-300 mg/day
D) 500-1000 mg/day

generally reserved for cases of treatment-resistant depression due to their side effect profile and dietary restrictions.

Answer: A) 20-40 mg/day

Explanation: The recommended dosage range for fluoxetine, a commonly prescribed SSRI for MDD, is 20-40 mg/day. However, dosages may vary depending on individual patient factors and treatment response.

DISRUPTIVE, IMPULSE-CONTROL, AND CONDUCT DISORDERS

Which of the following is characterized by a repetitive and persistent pattern of behavior that violates the rights of others and societal norms?
A) Conduct disorder
B) Antisocial personality disorder
C) Oppositional defiant disorder
D) Attention-deficit/hyperactivity disorder

Answer: A) Conduct disorder

Explanation: Conduct disorder is characterized by a repetitive and persistent pattern of behavior that violates the rights of others or societal norms. It involves aggression towards people and animals, destruction of property, deceitfulness, and serious rule violations.

How does conduct disorder differ from antisocial personality disorder (ASPD)?

Conduct disorder is typically diagnosed in childhood or adolescence, while ASPD is diagnosed in adulthood. Conduct disorder is typically diagnosed in childhood or adolescence, while antisocial personality disorder (ASPD) is diagnosed in adulthood. Conduct disorder is considered a precursor to ASPD, and individuals with conduct disorder are at higher risk of developing ASPD later in life.

Which of the following is a characteristic of oppositional defiant disorder (ODD)?
A) Aggression towards people and animals
B) Violation of societal norms and rights of others
C) Persistent pattern of angry/irritable mood
D) Persistent disregard for the safety of self or others

Answer: C) Persistent pattern of angry/irritable mood

Explanation: Oppositional defiant disorder (ODD) is characterized by a persistent pattern of angry or irritable mood, argumentative/defiant behavior, and vindictiveness. Unlike conduct disorder, ODD does not involve aggression towards people and animals or serious violations of societal norms.

Which of the following medications may be used in the treatment of conduct disorder?
A) Stimulants (e.g., methylphenidate)
B) Antipsychotics (e.g., risperidone)
C) Antidepressants (e.g., sertraline)
D) Mood stabilizers (e.g., lithium)

Answer: B) Antipsychotics (e.g., risperidone)

Explanation: Antipsychotic medications, such as risperidone, may be used in the treatment of conduct disorder when there are severe aggression and impulsive behaviors. These medications can help manage aggression and improve overall behavioral control.

Which laboratory test may be useful in assessing a patient with disruptive behavior disorders?
A) Thyroid function tests
B) Blood glucose levels
C) Toxicology screen
D) Serum iron levels

Answer: C) Toxicology screen

Explanation: Conduct disorder and other disruptive behavior disorders are not typically associated with specific laboratory abnormalities. However, a toxicology screen may be helpful to identify any substance abuse contributing to the disruptive behaviors.

Which aspect of health maintenance is important in the management of disruptive behavior disorders?

Regular therapy sessions and monitoring of treatment response

Explanation: Regular therapy sessions, such as cognitive-behavioral therapy or family therapy, are important in the management of disruptive behavior disorders. Monitoring treatment response and making necessary adjustments are crucial to improve behavioral outcomes and overall functioning.

Which eating disorder is characterized by self-imposed starvation, fear of weight gain, and distorted body image?
A) Anorexia nervosa
B) Bulimia nervosa
C) Binge eating disorder
D) Avoidant/restrictive food intake disorder

Answer: A) Anorexia nervosa

Explanation: Anorexia nervosa is characterized by self-imposed starvation, intense fear of weight gain, persistent restriction of food intake, and distorted body image. Individuals with anorexia nervosa often have an abnormally low body weight.

Which of the following is a characteristic of anorexia nervosa?
A) Recurrent episodes of binge eating
B) Compensatory behaviors, such as vomiting or excessive exercise
C) Persistent lack of interest in eating or food
D) Lanugo, a fine hair growth on the body

Answer: D) Lanugo, a fine hair growth on the body

Explanation: Lanugo is a fine hair growth that may develop on the body, including the face, arms, and back, in individuals with anorexia nervosa. It is an adaptive mechanism to help maintain body temperature due to the lack of body fat.

Which of the following is a characteristic of bulimia nervosa?
A) Intense fear of weight gain and body image distortion
B) Self-induced vomiting or misuse of laxatives/diuretics
C) Restricting food intake and avoiding eating in public
D) Excessive eating in a discrete period accompanied by a sense of lack of control

Answer: B) Self-induced vomiting or misuse of laxatives/diuretics

Explanation: Bulimia nervosa is characterized by recurrent episodes of binge eating followed by compensatory behaviors, such as self-induced vomiting or misuse of laxatives/diuretics. The person often feels a lack of control during the binge-eating episodes.

What physical examination finding is associated with repeated self-induced vomiting in bulimia nervosa?
A) Lanugo
B) Russel sign
C) Bradycardia
D) Hypotension

Answer: B) Russel sign

Explanation: Russel sign refers to the presence of calluses or scars on the knuckles or back of the hand. It is associated with repeated self-induced vomiting, where the hand is used to induce gag reflex. It is commonly observed in individuals with bulimia nervosa. Lanugo is more so associated with anorexia nervosa. This question was specifically asking about bulimia nervosa.

What is the first-line treatment for anorexia nervosa?
A) Cognitive-behavioral therapy (CBT)
B) Antidepressant medications
C) Nutritional rehabilitation and weight restoration
D) Family-based therapy (FBT)

Answer: C) Nutritional rehabilitation and weight restoration

Explanation: The initial focus in treating anorexia nervosa is nutritional rehabilitation and weight restoration. This includes addressing malnutrition, establishing regular eating patterns, and achieving a healthy weight. Psychotherapy, such as cognitive-behavioral therapy (CBT) or family-based therapy (FBT), is often combined with nutritional rehabilitation.

Which laboratory finding is commonly seen in individuals with anorexia nervosa?

Answer: B) Hypokalemia (low potassium levels)

A) Elevated blood glucose levels
B) Hypokalemia (low potassium levels)
C) Increased hemoglobin levels
D) Elevated cholesterol levels

What is the primary goal of treatment for bulimia nervosa?
A) Achieving weight restoration
B) Normalizing eating patterns and reducing binge-purge behaviors
C) Addressing body image distortion and improving self-esteem
D) Treating comorbid psychiatric conditions

Which of the following is a medication that may be used in the treatment of bulimia nervosa?
A) Fluoxetine (Prozac)
B) Bupropion (Wellbutrin)
C) Risperidone (Risperdal)
D) Diazepam (Valium)

What is the most common cause of death in individuals with eating disorders?
A) Cardiac arrhythmias
B) Suicide
C) Malnutrition
D) Gastrointestinal complications

Explanation: Hypokalemia is commonly seen in individuals with anorexia nervosa due to inadequate intake of potassium-rich foods and purging behaviors. It can lead to various complications, including cardiac arrhythmias and muscle weakness.

Answer: B) Normalizing eating patterns and reducing binge-purge behaviors

Explanation: The primary goal of treatment for bulimia nervosa is to normalize eating patterns and reduce binge-purge behaviors. This involves psychotherapy, such as cognitive-behavioral therapy (CBT), to address the underlying psychological factors contributing to the disorder.

Answer: A) Fluoxetine (Prozac)

Explanation: Fluoxetine, a selective serotonin reuptake inhibitor (SSRI), is the only medication approved by the FDA for the treatment of bulimia nervosa. It can help reduce binge-eating episodes and improve mood symptoms.

Answer: B) Suicide

Explanation: While various complications can arise from eating disorders, including cardiac abnormalities and malnutrition, suicide is the most common cause of death in individuals with eating disorders. It underscores the importance of early detection, intervention, and appropriate mental health support.

What is the most common risk factor for suicide?

A history of previous suicide attempts is the most common risk factor for suicide.

What are the signs and symptoms of those who may be at risk for suicide?

1. Expressing thoughts of suicide or a desire to die.
2. Withdrawing from social activities and isolating oneself.
3. Drastic mood swings, including extreme sadness and sudden calmness.
4. Giving away possessions or making statements implying not needing them.
5. Increased substance abuse.
6. Changes in sleep patterns, such as insomnia or excessive sleeping.
7. Engaging in reckless behavior without concern for personal safety.
8. Expressing feelings of being a burden to others.
9. Sudden improvement in mood after a period of depression.

What is the most common type of therapy used in the treatment of suicidal individuals?

Cognitive-Behavioral Therapy (CBT) is the most common type of therapy used in the treatment of suicidal individuals.

Which of the following medications can be used in the treatment of depression and suicidal ideation?
A) Benzodiazepines

Answer: C) Selective serotonin reuptake inhibitors (SSRIs)

B) Antipsychotics
C) Selective serotonin reuptake inhibitors (SSRIs)
D) Opioids

AVASCULAR NECROSIS OF THE FEMORAL HEAD

What is the other term to describe avascular necrosis of the femoral head seen in the adolescent population?	Legg-Calve-Perthes disease
What is one unique finding on physical exam for Legg-Calve-Perthes disease?	Decreased internal rotation of the affected hip, radiating pain to the ipsilateral knee, dull pain
What it the typical age range seen in Legg-Calve-Perthes disease	Ages 4-10 years old
What is the best initial test to diagnose Legg-Calve-Perthes disease?	X-ray
What is the best confirmatory test to diagnose Legg-Calve-Perthes disease?	MRI
What is the treatment for Legg-Calve-Perthes disease?	May be conservative. If aggressive—joint replacement.

CONGENITAL HIP DYSPLASIA

What is congenital hip dysplasia?	Hip instability, subluxation/dislocation of the femoral head
What are signs and symptoms of congenital hip dysplasia?	Unequal/asymmetric thigh folds, shortening of the leg. May develop limping and waddling gait
What are the two physical exam maneuvers that can be performed for congenital hip dysplasia?	Barlow and Ortolani
How do you perform the Barlow and Ortolani maneuvers?	Barlow—adduct the hips and apply a force posteriorly. Ortolani—abduct the hips and apply force in the anterior direction (e.g., reduce the hip if dislocated from the Barlow maneuver)
What is seen on physical exam in the work up of congenital hip dysplasia?	Limited hip abduction. + Galeazzi (e.g., unequal knee height compared b/l), + Barlow (e.g., palpable clunk felt by hip dislocation when the hip is flexed and adducted and a downward pressure is applied to the infant), + Ortolani (e.g., palpable clunk felt by hip reduction when the hip is flexed, abducted, and an upward pressure is applied)
What is the treatment for < 6 months old?	Pavlik harness
What is the treatment for 6-18 months old?	Closed reduction -> immobilization with hip spica cast
What is the treatment for > 18 months old?	Surgical therapy

JUVENILE RHEUMATOID ARTHRITIS (RA)

What is the most common presenting symptom of juvenile rheumatoid arthritis (JRA)?	Answer: Joint pain and swelling. Explanation: Joint pain and swelling are the most common presenting symptoms of JRA. Children may experience stiffness, limited range of motion, and joint tenderness. Other symptoms may include fatigue, low-grade fever, and rash. JRA is characterized by chronic arthritis in children under the age of 16, lasting for at least six weeks.
What is the most common type of juvenile RA?	Oligoarticular
What age is the onset for juvenile RA?	Younger than 16-years-old

What are the signs and symptoms for juvenile RA?	Arthritis, generalized adenopathy, splenomegaly, fever, or unexplained rash.
Which labs do you order in the workup of juvenile RA?	CBC, CMP, ESR, CRP, ANA, RF, anti-CCP, and HLA-B27
What is the diagnostic criterion for JRA?	Answer: Arthritis in one or more joints for at least six weeks in a child under the age of 16. Explanation: The diagnostic criterion for JRA is the presence of arthritis in one or more joints for at least six weeks in a child under the age of 16. The arthritis should not be attributable to any other known cause.
Which imaging modality may be helpful in assessing joint damage in JRA?	Answer: Radiographs (X-rays). Explanation: Radiographs (X-rays) may be helpful in assessing joint damage in JRA. They can show joint space narrowing, erosions, and bony changes associated with chronic inflammation.
What is the first-line treatment for JRA?	Answer: Nonsteroidal anti-inflammatory drugs (NSAIDs) and physical therapy. Explanation: Nonsteroidal anti-inflammatory drugs (NSAIDs), such as ibuprofen or naproxen, are commonly used as first-line treatment to reduce pain and inflammation in JRA. Physical therapy is also an important component of treatment to maintain joint mobility and strength.
Which medication is considered the mainstay of JRA treatment for more severe cases?	Answer: Disease-modifying antirheumatic drugs (DMARDs), such as methotrexate. Explanation: In more severe cases of JRA, disease-modifying antirheumatic drugs (DMARDs), such as methotrexate, are considered the mainstay of treatment. DMARDs help to control inflammation and slow down the progression of joint damage.
What is the role of corticosteroids in the treatment of JRA?	Answer: Corticosteroids are used to control severe symptoms and reduce inflammation but are generally reserved for short-term use due to potential side effects. Explanation: Corticosteroids may be used in JRA to control severe symptoms and reduce inflammation. However, they are generally reserved for short-term use due to potential side effects, such as growth delay and increased susceptibility to infections.

NEOPLASMS OF THE MUSCULOSKELETAL SYSTEM

A 16-year-old female presents with a painful mass on her left forearm. On physical examination, there is a small, mobile, subcutaneous nodule. Radiographs show a well-defined lesion with stippled calcifications. Laboratory tests reveal elevated serum calcium levels. What is the most likely diagnosis? **A) Osteosarcoma**	Explanation: The most likely diagnosis in this case is osteoid osteoma (Option B). Osteoid osteoma is a benign bone tumor that commonly presents with localized pain that is worse at night and is relieved by aspirin or nonsteroidal anti-inflammatory drugs (NSAIDs). On physical examination, a small, mobile, subcutaneous nodule may be palpated. Radiographically, osteoid osteomas typically

B) Osteoid osteoma
C) Lipoma
D) Myositis ossificans
E) Chondrosarcoma

A 12-year-old male presents with pain and swelling in his left leg. Imaging reveals a diaphyseal lesion with onion-skin appearance, periosteal reaction, and a soft tissue mass. Biopsy shows small round blue cells and a positive EWSR1 gene rearrangement. What is the most likely diagnosis?
A) Osteosarcoma
B) Ewing sarcoma
C) Chondrosarcoma
D) Osteochondroma
E) Giant cell tumor

A 25-year-old female presents with a painless, bony, hard mass on her proximal humerus. Imaging reveals a pedunculated lesion with a cartilage cap. The lesion is continuous with the underlying bone. What is the most likely diagnosis?
A) Osteosarcoma
B) Ewing sarcoma
C) Chondrosarcoma
D) Osteochondroma
E) Giant cell tumor

A 16-year-old male presents with pain and swelling in his right knee for the past few months. On physical examination, there is a palpable mass over the distal femur. Radiographs show a sunburst pattern and Codman triangle. Which of the following is the most appropriate next step in the diagnosis of this patient?
A) Fine-needle aspiration biopsy
B) Core needle biopsy
C) Surgical excisional biopsy
D) MRI of the affected area
E) Plain radiographs of the chest

demonstrate a well-defined lesion with stippled calcifications, known as the "nidus." Lipoma (Option C) is a benign soft tissue tumor and would not show stippled calcifications on radiographs. Myositis ossificans (Option D) is the formation of heterotopic bone within muscle tissue, usually as a result of trauma, and would not present as a subcutaneous nodule. Osteosarcoma (Option A) is a primary malignant bone tumor and would not typically present as a small, subcutaneous nodule. Chondrosarcoma (Option E) arises from cartilage and would not demonstrate stippled calcifications on radiographs.
Explanation: The most likely diagnosis in this case is Ewing sarcoma (Option B). Ewing sarcoma is a malignant bone tumor that commonly affects children and young adults. It typically presents with pain, swelling, and a soft tissue mass. Radiographically, Ewing sarcoma may show a diaphyseal lesion with an onion-skin appearance and periosteal reaction. Histologically, it is characterized by small round blue cells. The presence of a positive EWSR1 gene rearrangement is a defining feature of Ewing sarcoma.

Explanation: The most likely diagnosis in this case is osteochondroma (Option D). Osteochondroma is a benign bone tumor characterized by an overgrowth of cartilage-capped bone projecting from the surface. It commonly occurs in the long bones, such as the proximal humerus, and typically presents as a painless, bony mass. Radiographically, osteochondromas are pedunculated lesions with a cartilage cap that is continuous with the underlying bone.

Explanation: The most appropriate next step in the diagnosis of this patient is core needle biopsy (Option B). Osteosarcoma is a malignant bone tumor commonly seen in children and adolescents. It typically presents with pain, swelling, and a palpable mass. Radiographically, osteosarcoma often shows a sunburst pattern and Codman triangle. To confirm the diagnosis, a tissue sample should be obtained for histopathological examination. Core needle biopsy is the preferred method as it provides an adequate sample for diagnosis while minimizing the risk of tumor seeding. Fine-needle aspiration biopsy (Option A) may not provide enough tissue for a definitive diagnosis. Surgical excisional biopsy (Option C) is not typically performed for suspected osteosarcoma due to the risk of tumor dissemination. MRI (Option D) is useful for evaluating the extent of disease, but biopsy is required for a definitive diagnosis. Plain radiographs of the chest (Option E) are necessary to evaluate for the presence of pulmonary metastases, which are common in osteosarcoma, but biopsy should be performed first.

What is nursemaid elbow?	Radial head subluxation/dislocation
What is the classic presentation of nursemaid elbow?	Caretaker swinging child by arm which causes a "pulled elbow"
Which ligament is affected in nursemaid elbow?	Annular ligament displacement
What are the signs and symptoms of nursemaid elbow?	Pain, tenderness, limited ROM, guarding, arm held in flexion and pronation (e.g., inability to supinate forearm); patient will resist forearm PROM
What are the two techniques to reduce the displaced elbow seen in nursemaid elbow?	Hyperpronation OR supination followed by flexion of the elbow
Which of the following is the preferred method in the reduction of a radial head subluxation on the first attempt?	Hyperpronation of the forearm > supination and flexion on the first attempted attempt

OSGOOD-SCHLATTER DISEASE

What is Osgood-Schlatter disease?	Traction of the apophysitis of the tibial tubercle during adolescent growth spurts
Osgood-Schlatter disease commonly affects which age and population?	Young, active adolescent boys aged 10-15
What are the signs and symptoms of Osgood-Schlatter disease?	Tenderness over the tibial tuberosity, pain that is worse with flexion or running.
What is the treatment for Osgood-Schlatter disease?	Rest, ice, stretching. Pain medications (e.g., NSAIDs or acetaminophen)

SCOLIOSIS

What is scoliosis?	Scoliosis is a lateral curvature of the spine greater than 10 degrees, often accompanied by vertebral rotation.
How is the degree of scoliosis measured?	The degree of scoliosis is measured using the Cobb angle, which assesses the angle between the most tilted vertebrae at the apex of the curve.

A 14-year-old female presents to the clinic for a routine check-up. On physical examination, you notice asymmetry of the shoulders, prominence of the right scapula, and an apparent rib hump on forward bending. The patient denies any pain or discomfort. Upon further evaluation, you measure the Cobb angle on an X-ray of the spine and find it to be 32 degrees. Based on the clinical findings and Cobb angle measurement, which of the following is the most appropriate management for this patient?
A) Observation with regular follow-up every 6 months
B) Prescription of a thoracolumbosacral orthosis (TLSO)
C) Referral to a pediatric orthopedic surgeon for surgical evaluation
D) Prescribing exercises for postural correction

Answer:
A) Observation with regular follow-up every 6 months

Explanation:
In this patient with clinical signs of scoliosis and a Cobb angle measurement of 32 degrees, the most appropriate initial management is observation with regular follow-up every 6 months. The recommended management approach for idiopathic scoliosis is primarily based on the degree of the Cobb angle and the patient's age. In adolescents with a Cobb angle less than 25-30 degrees and no evidence of progression, observation with regular follow-up is typically indicated. This allows monitoring for any progression of the curvature and appropriate intervention if necessary. Prescription of a thoracolumbosacral orthosis (TLSO) is reserved for moderate curves (25-40 degrees) with documented progression or in cases where observation alone is insufficient. Referral to a pediatric orthopedic surgeon for surgical evaluation is typically reserved for severe curves (greater than 40-45 degrees) or if the curve is rapidly progressing. Prescribing exercises for postural correction can be beneficial in mild cases but are not the primary management strategy. Therefore, the correct answer is A) Observation with regular follow-up every 6 months.

What is the name of the physical exam maneuver to routinely assess for scoliosis in adolescents?	Adams forward test
What is the primary treatment for scoliosis with documented progression?	Brace (orthosis) treatment is the primary non-surgical intervention for scoliosis in moderate curves (25-40 degrees) with documented progression. The most common type is the thoracolumbosacral orthosis (TLSO), which helps prevent further curvature progression during skeletal growth.
When is surgical intervention considered for scoliosis?	Surgical intervention is considered for severe scoliosis (greater than 40-45 degrees) or rapidly progressing curves. Spinal fusion with instrumentation is the most common surgical procedure performed, aiming to correct and stabilize the curvature.

What is slipped capital femoral epiphysis (SCFE)?	SCFE is a condition in which the growth plate at the head of the femur (thighbone) becomes weak and the ball at the head of the femur slips off the neck of the bone.
What are the risk factors for SCFE?	Obesity, adolescence, M > F
What is the pathophysiological mechanism for which a SCFE occurs?	Shearing at the proximal femoral physis -> weakens and leads to an anterosuperior displacement of the proximal femur diaphysis (e.g., gives the appearance of a posteriorly displaced femoral head)
What is the most common age group affected by SCFE?	SCFE most commonly affects children and adolescents between the ages of 10 and 16 years.
What are the signs and symptoms of SCFE?	Hip or knee pain, limp or inability to bear weight on the affected leg, restricted hip motion, and outward rotation of the leg.
A 13-year-old overweight male presents to the clinic with a complaint of left hip and knee pain for the past several weeks. He reports a noticeable limp and difficulty walking. On physical examination, there is limited internal rotation of the left hip with external rotation of the leg. The patient denies any recent trauma or injury. X-ray of the left hip reveals a slipped capital femoral epiphysis. What is the most appropriate initial management for this patient's condition? **A) Prescribe non-steroidal anti-inflammatory drugs (NSAIDs) for pain relief** **B) Recommend immediate weight-bearing on the affected leg** **C) Administer intravenous antibiotics to prevent infection** **D) Refer the patient for urgent surgical intervention**	Answer: D) Refer the patient for urgent surgical intervention Explanation: The most appropriate initial management for this patient with a confirmed diagnosis of slipped capital femoral epiphysis (SCFE) is to refer the patient for urgent surgical intervention. SCFE is a medical emergency that requires prompt stabilization of the hip joint to prevent further slippage and minimize the risk of complications, such as avascular necrosis. Surgical intervention typically involves the placement of screws or pins to stabilize the femoral head and neck. Non-steroidal anti-inflammatory drugs (NSAIDs) may be used for pain relief, but they do not address the underlying issue and are not the primary management strategy. Weight-bearing on the affected leg should be restricted to prevent additional damage. Intravenous antibiotics are not indicated unless there is evidence of infection or complications such as a concurrent septic hip. Therefore, the correct answer is D) Refer the patient for urgent surgical intervention.

DIABETES MELLITUS

Which is more prevalent, diabetes mellitus type 1 or type 2?

Diabetes mellitus type 2 is more prevalent (about 90% of all diabetes mellitus cases)

What does HbA1c measure and how is it used in diabetes management?
A) HbA1c measures fasting blood glucose levels.
B) HbA1c measures average blood glucose levels over the past 2-3 months.
C) HbA1c measures insulin resistance.
D) HbA1c measures postprandial blood glucose levels.

Answer: B) HbA1c measures average blood glucose levels over the past 2-3 months.

Explanation: HbA1c (hemoglobin A1c) is a blood test that reflects average blood glucose levels over the past 2-3 months. It is used to assess long-term glycemic control in individuals with diabetes. A lower HbA1c value indicates better blood glucose control, while higher values indicate poorer control and may necessitate adjustments in medication, diet, or lifestyle.

Incorrect choices:
A) HbA1c is not a measure of fasting blood glucose levels, but rather a reflection of average blood glucose levels over time.
C) HbA1c does not measure insulin resistance directly but rather provides an assessment of overall glycemic control.
D) HbA1c does not specifically measure postprandial blood glucose levels but provides an average of blood glucose levels over a longer time period.

What is diabetes mellitus type 1?

Insulin deficiency due to pancreatic beta cell destruction

What is the main difference between type 1 diabetes mellitus and type 2 diabetes mellitus?

Type 1 diabetes is an autoimmune condition characterized by the destruction of pancreatic beta cells, resulting in absolute insulin deficiency. Type 2 diabetes is primarily due to insulin resistance and impaired insulin secretion.

Explanation: Type 1 diabetes mellitus is an autoimmune disorder in which the immune system mistakenly attacks and destroys the insulin-producing beta cells in the pancreas. As a result, individuals with type 1 diabetes lack insulin production and require lifelong insulin replacement therapy. Type 2 diabetes mellitus, on the other hand, is primarily caused by insulin resistance, where the body's cells do not respond effectively to insulin. This leads to elevated blood glucose levels. Additionally, type 2 diabetes involves impaired insulin secretion from the pancreas.

What is the dawn phenomenon?

Glucose rises the most through the early hours (e.g., 2am-8am).

How do you treat dawn phenomenon?

Bedtime long-acting insulin

What is the Somogyi effect?

Nocturnal hypoglycemia followed by rebound hyperglycemia

What is diabetic ketoacidosis (DKA)?

Diabetic ketoacidosis is a life-threatening complication primarily seen in individuals with type 1 diabetes, characterized by severe hyperglycemia, ketosis, and metabolic acidosis.

Explanation: Diabetic ketoacidosis occurs when there is a severe lack of insulin in the body, resulting in the inability of cells to use glucose for energy. In response, the body breaks down fats as an alternative energy source, leading to the production of ketones. Elevated ketone levels cause metabolic acidosis, resulting in a decrease in blood pH. DKA is characterized by symptoms such as excessive thirst, frequent urination, abdominal pain, nausea, vomiting, fruity breath odor, and altered mental status. Immediate medical attention and intravenous insulin therapy are required to treat DKA.

What is the presentation for DKA?

Fruity breath, tachypnea, tachycardia, hypotension, and Kussmaul breathing

What do the labs show for DKA?

Plasma glucose > 250, pH < 7.3, serum bicarbonate < 15 mEq/L, (+) ketones in urine and serum

How do you treat DKA?

IV fluids, insulin, and potassium

What are the risk factors for developing type 2 diabetes mellitus?

Risk factors for type 2 diabetes include obesity, sedentary lifestyle, family history, older age, and certain ethnic backgrounds.

What are the signs and symptoms of T2DM?

Polyuria, polydipsia, nocturia. Acanthosis nigricans is a sign of insulin resistance

What are the diagnostics of T2DM?

Fasting serum glucose ≥ 126 mg/dL on 2 separate occasions OR **2-hour glucose value after OGTT of ≥ 200 mg/dL** OR **RBG of ≥ 200 mg/dL with symptoms** OR **HbA1C of ≥ 6.5%**

What are some oral medications commonly used in the treatment of type 2 diabetes?

Oral medications for type 2 diabetes include metformin, sulfonylureas, DPP-4 inhibitors, SGLT-2 inhibitors, and thiazolidinediones.

Explanation: There are several classes of oral medications used in the treatment of type 2 diabetes. Metformin is often the first-line medication and works by reducing glucose production in the liver and improving insulin sensitivity. Sulfonylureas stimulate insulin release from the pancreas. DPP-4 inhibitors, SGLT-2 inhibitors, and thiazolidinediones work through different mechanisms to help manage blood glucose levels.

Which medication class stimulates insulin release from pancreatic beta cells and may cause hypoglycemia?

Answer: Sulfonylureas

Explanation: Sulfonylureas are a class of oral antidiabetic medications that work by stimulating insulin release from pancreatic beta cells. They act by closing ATP-dependent potassium channels on the beta cell membrane, leading to depolarization and subsequent release of insulin. However, sulfonylureas can sometimes lead to hypoglycemia, particularly if taken in excessive doses or if meal timing is irregular.

What is GLP-1 receptor agonist (GLP-1RA) and how does it work in diabetes management?

GLP-1 receptor agonists are injectable medications used in the treatment of type 2 diabetes. They mimic the effects of the hormone GLP-1 and promote insulin release, inhibit glucagon secretion, slow gastric emptying, and promote satiety.

Explanation: GLP-1 receptor agonists, such as exenatide

HYPERCALCEMIA	
What is hypercalcemia?	Hypercalcemia is a condition characterized by elevated levels of calcium in the blood.

Explanation: Hypercalcemia refers to higher-than-normal levels of calcium in the bloodstream. Normal calcium levels range from 8.5 to 10.5 mg/dL. Hypercalcemia can result from various underlying causes, such as overactive parathyroid glands, certain cancers, medications, or underlying medical conditions.

What are the common symptoms of hypercalcemia?
Symptoms of hypercalcemia can include fatigue, thirst, constipation, nausea, bone pain, and confusion.

Explanation: Hypercalcemia can cause a range of symptoms, including fatigue, excessive thirst, constipation, nausea, bone pain, frequent urination, kidney stones, and confusion. The severity of symptoms can vary depending on the degree of calcium elevation and the underlying cause.

What is the primary hormone involved in regulating calcium levels in the blood?
Parathyroid hormone (PTH) is the primary hormone involved in regulating calcium levels.

Explanation: Parathyroid hormone (PTH) is produced by the parathyroid glands and plays a key role in maintaining calcium homeostasis. When blood calcium levels are low, PTH is released, promoting the release of calcium from bones, reabsorption of calcium in the kidneys, and increased absorption of calcium in the intestines. In hypercalcemia, there may be overactivity of the parathyroid glands, leading to excessive calcium release.

What is the main role of calcitonin in calcium regulation?
A) Promotion of calcium release from bones
B) Enhancement of calcium absorption in the intestines
C) Inhibition of calcium reabsorption in the kidneys
D) Stimulation of parathyroid hormone (PTH) release
C) Inhibition of calcium reabsorption in the kidneys

Explanation: Calcitonin is a hormone produced by the thyroid gland. Its primary role is to inhibit calcium reabsorption in the kidneys, leading to increased urinary excretion of calcium. This helps to lower blood calcium levels and counteract the effects of parathyroid hormone (PTH), which promotes calcium release from bones.

Incorrect choices:
A) Calcitonin does not promote calcium release from bones. In fact, it works in opposition to parathyroid hormone (PTH) to lower blood calcium levels.
B) Calcium absorption in the intestines is primarily regulated by vitamin D, not calcitonin.
D) Calcitonin does not stimulate the release of parathyroid hormone (PTH). Rather, it has an opposing

How is hypercalcemia diagnosed?

effect to PTH, helping to maintain calcium homeostasis.

Hypercalcemia is diagnosed through blood tests, primarily measuring serum calcium levels and assessing PTH levels.

Explanation: The diagnosis of hypercalcemia is typically made by measuring serum calcium levels. If hypercalcemia is present, further testing may be done to determine the underlying cause. This may include measuring PTH levels, as well as evaluating other parameters such as vitamin D levels, kidney function, and imaging studies (e.g., X-ray, bone scan) to identify any bone abnormalities or potential malignancies.

What are the treatment options for hypercalcemia?

The treatment of hypercalcemia depends on the underlying cause and may involve hydration, medications (such as bisphosphonates or calcitonin), and addressing the underlying condition.

Explanation: Treatment of hypercalcemia aims to lower blood calcium levels and address the underlying cause. Hydration is often an initial step to help increase urinary calcium excretion. Medications like bisphosphonates or calcitonin may be used to inhibit bone resorption and reduce calcium levels. Additionally, treating the underlying condition, such as addressing overactive parathyroid glands or managing cancer-related hypercalcemia, is essential to achieve long-term control.

Which of the following laboratory abnormalities may be seen in hypercalcemia?
A) Hyperphosphatemia
B) Hypokalemia
C) Hyponatremia
D) Hypoglycemia

Answer: A) Hyperphosphatemia

Explanation: Hypercalcemia can disrupt the balance of other electrolytes in the body. One common finding is hyperphosphatemia, characterized by an elevation in serum phosphate levels. This occurs due to increased renal reabsorption of phosphate as a compensatory mechanism for the elevated calcium levels.

Incorrect choices:
B) Hypokalemia refers to low levels of potassium in the blood and is not typically associated with hypercalcemia.
C) Hyponatremia indicates low levels of sodium in the blood and is not directly related to hypercalcemia.
D) Hypoglycemia refers to low blood glucose levels and is unrelated to hypercalcemia.

HYPERTHYROIDISM

What is hyperthyroidism?

Metabolic overdrive due to overproduction of the T4 and T3 thyroid hormones

What is the most common cause of hyperthyroidism?

Grave's disease

What are the signs and symptoms of hyperthyroidism?

Tachycardia, palpitations, heat intolerance, weight loss, hyperactivity, fatigue, nervous, insomnia

What are the signs and symptoms of Grave's disease?	Pretibial myxedema, proptosis (e.g., exophthalmos), and lid lag
What is seen on labs in the workup of hyperthyroidism?	Decreased TSH, increased free T4 and increased total T3, and increased uptake of radioactive iodine (seen in Grave's—Autoantibody tests (e.g., TSH receptor antibody, antithyroid peroxidase Ab and anti-Tg antibodies)
What is the treatment for hyperthyroidism?	Methimazole or PTU (for pregnancy). Symptomatic relief—beta blocker (e.g., propranolol)

HYPOTHYROIDISM

What is hypothyroidism?	A condition in which the thyroid gland is underactive resulting in low thyroid hormone
What is the most common cause of juvenile hypothyroidism?	Hashimoto thyroiditis
What labs are seen in the diagnosis of Hashimoto thyroiditis?	(+) antithyroid peroxidase and anti-thyroglobulin antibodies
What are the signs and symptoms of hypothyroidism?	Dry, brittle hair, excessive fatigue, cool, dry skin, intolerance to cold, bradycardia, constipation, weight gain, secondary amenorrhea, muscle cramps, hyporeflexia, myxedema.
What is congenital hypothyroidism?	A condition that is generally asymptomatic at birth but can later develop into classic hypothyroidism-like symptoms
How is congenital hypothyroidism diagnosed?	Identified through neonatal screening
What is another name for congenital hypothyroidism?	Cretinism
What is the presentation for congenital hypothyroidism?	Round face, lethargy, protruding tongue, hoarse cry, distended abdomen, dry skin, hypotonia, hypothermia, poor weight gain, poor feeding, and constipation
What labs are seen in the workup of hypothyroidism?	Best initial test—serum TSH elevated. Confirmatory—low free T4. Serum thyroid antibody testing—thyroglobulin antibodies and thyroid peroxidase antibodies—detectable in majority of autoimmune hypothyroidism cases; TSH receptor antibodies detectable in 20% of autoimmune hypothyroidism
What is the treatment for hypothyroidism?	Levothyroxine

OBESITY

What is the criteria for diagnosing BMI in the pediatric population?	BMI in the 95th percentile or higher for age and sex
Being overweight is between which range of BMI percentile?	Overweight = BMI between 85-94th percentile
What is metabolic syndrome?	HDL < 40mg/dL in males or < 50 mg/dL in females, BP > 135/85 mmHg, TG > 150 mg/dL, waist circumference > 35 in in females or > 40 inches for males, or increased fasting blood glucose or two-hour oral glucose tolerance test
Which treatment is first-line for metabolic syndrome?	Non-pharm—lifestyle modification. Pharm—metformin
What is the recommended screening for a 10-year-old in the 50th percentile for BMI?	Fasting lipid screening
	Between ages 9-11- or 18–21-year-old and in the 5th-84th percentile, a fasting lipid panel is recommended routinely

| **What is the recommended screening for a 15-year-old in the 95th percentile?** | Dyslipidemia—order fasting lipid panel, check fasting glucose if concerns for T2DM OR check HbA1C, check liver function levels—alanine transaminase levels, check blood pressure, measure waist circumference |
| **What are recommended patient education points for patients diagnosed with obesity?** | Recommended increased intake of fruits and vegetables, limited screen time (e.g., TV, pads, computers, video games), minimize juice and other sweetened beverages, eat breakfast (don't skip), 30 minutes to one hour of physical activity each day (set realistic goals), engage family and encourage group activities |

SHORT STATURE

What is another name for short stature?	Dwarfism
What is the definition of short stature?	2 standard deviations below the mean for children of the same sex and chronological age
At which age is puberty considered delayed?	No secondary sex characteristics by age 14 in males and 12 in females
What is the most common cause of short stature?	Familial (genetic) short stature and constitutional short stature
What is the best test to order if you are concerned about height and weight percentiles from the growth chart?	Check bone age by ordering an AP x-ray of the hand

ANEMIA

What is anemia?

Anemia is a condition characterized by a decrease in the number of red blood cells or a decrease in the amount of hemoglobin in the blood.

What are the common symptoms of anemia?

Common symptoms of anemia include fatigue, weakness, shortness of breath, pale skin, dizziness, and rapid or irregular heartbeat.

Explanation: These symptoms occur due to the decreased oxygen-carrying capacity of the blood.

What is the most common cause of anemia worldwide?

Iron deficiency anemia is the most common cause of anemia globally.

Explanation: Iron deficiency can occur due to inadequate dietary intake, poor absorption, increased iron requirements (e.g., during pregnancy), or chronic blood loss.

Which lab test is typically used to diagnose anemia?

Complete Blood Count (CBC) is commonly used to diagnose anemia.

Explanation: CBC measures the levels of red blood cells, hemoglobin, hematocrit, and other parameters that help in evaluating the type and severity of anemia.

What is the normal range of hemoglobin in adult males and females?
a) Males: 13.5-17.5 g/dL
b) Females: 12.0-15.5 g/dL
c) Males: 14.0-18.0 g/dL
d) Females: 11.0-14.0 g/dL

The correct answer is (c). These ranges represent the normal values for hemoglobin in adult males and females.

Reasoning: Answer (a) is incorrect because the given range is slightly lower than the normal values. Answer (b) is incorrect because the given range is slightly lower for males and slightly higher for females. Answer (d) is incorrect because the given range is lower than the normal values for both males and females.

What is the treatment of choice for megaloblastic anemia?

Megaloblastic anemia is treated with vitamin B12 and/or folate supplementation.

Explanation: Megaloblastic anemia results from deficiencies of vitamin B12 or folate, and treatment involves correcting the underlying deficiency.

Which of the following is not a type of anemia?
a) Aplastic anemia
b) Hemophilia
c) Thalassemia
d) Pernicious anemia

The correct answer is (b), Hemophilia.

Reasoning: Hemophilia is a bleeding disorder caused by a deficiency or dysfunction of clotting factors, not a type of anemia. Aplastic anemia (a) is characterized by a decrease in the production of all blood cells. Thalassemia (c) is a group of genetic disorders affecting hemoglobin production. Pernicious anemia (d) is a type of megaloblastic anemia caused by vitamin B12 deficiency.

What is the most common inherited bleeding disorder?

Von Willebrand disease is the most common inherited bleeding disorder.

Explanation: Von Willebrand disease is caused by a deficiency or dysfunction of von Willebrand factor, which plays a crucial role in platelet function and clotting.

Which vitamin is essential for the synthesis of clotting factors II, VII, IX, and X?
a) Vitamin C
b) Vitamin K
c) Vitamin D
d) Vitamin B12

The correct answer is (b), Vitamin K.

Reasoning: Vitamin K is essential for the synthesis of clotting factors II, VII, IX, and X. Vitamin C (a) is involved in collagen synthesis, Vitamin D (c) regulates calcium metabolism, and Vitamin B12 (d) is necessary for red blood cell production.

What is the treatment of choice for hemophilia A?

The treatment of choice for hemophilia A is replacement therapy with factor VIII.

Explanation: Hemophilia A is caused by a deficiency or dysfunction of factor VIII, and replacing the missing factor VIII is the mainstay of treatment.

Which of the following is not a symptom of thrombocytopenia?
a) Easy bruising
b) Prolonged bleeding after injury
c) Petechiae
d) Iron deficiency

The correct answer is (d), Iron deficiency.

Reasoning: Thrombocytopenia is characterized by a low platelet count and can manifest as easy bruising (a), prolonged bleeding after injury (b), and the presence of petechiae (c). Iron deficiency (d) is not directly related to thrombocytopenia.

Which medication is commonly used to prevent blood clot formation in patients with inherited thrombophilias?

Anticoagulant medications such as warfarin or direct oral anticoagulants (DOACs) are commonly used to prevent blood clot formation in patients with inherited thrombophilias.

Explanation: Inherited thrombophilias are genetic conditions that increase the risk of blood clot formation, and anticoagulant medications help prevent clotting.

Which condition is characterized by spontaneous, recurrent episodes of bleeding into joints and muscles?

Hemophilia is characterized by spontaneous, recurrent episodes of bleeding into joints and muscles.

Explanation: Hemophilia is a genetic bleeding disorder, primarily affecting males, and is characterized by a deficiency or dysfunction of clotting factors, leading to prolonged bleeding and spontaneous bleeding episodes.

Which pediatric brain tumor arises from the cerebellum?

Medulloblastoma
Explanation: Medulloblastoma is a type of brain tumor that arises in the cerebellum, which is responsible for coordination and balance. It is the most common malignant brain tumor in children. Medulloblastomas can cause symptoms such as headaches, nausea, and

Which pediatric brain tumor is commonly associated with the genetic disorder neurofibromatosis type 1?

problems with motor skills due to their location in the posterior fossa of the brain.

Astrocytomas can be associated with neurofibromatosis type 1 (NF1), a genetic disorder characterized by multiple neurofibromas and café-au-lait spots. Children with NF1 have an increased risk of developing astrocytomas, particularly optic pathway gliomas, which can affect the optic nerves and cause visual problems.

Which pediatric brain tumor arises from the cells lining the ventricles of the brain?

Ependymoma.

Explanation: Ependymomas originate from the ependymal cells that line the ventricles of the brain and the central canal of the spinal cord. These tumors commonly occur in children and can cause symptoms such as hydrocephalus due to obstruction of cerebrospinal fluid flow within the ventricles.

A 6-month-old infant is brought to the pediatrician by concerned parents who have noticed a persistent squint (strabismus) in the child's right eye. On examination, the right eye deviates inward (esotropia) consistently. The red reflex is normal bilaterally. There are no other abnormal findings on physical examination. The child has no significant past medical history, and there is no family history of eye conditions or cancers. What is the most likely diagnosis in this patient?
A) Congenital cataract
B) Retinoblastoma
C) Amblyopia
D) Duane syndrome

Answer: B) Retinoblastoma

Explanation: The presence of a persistent squint (strabismus), specifically inward deviation of the eye (esotropia), in a young child is a concerning sign for retinoblastoma. Strabismus in retinoblastoma occurs due to the tumor's growth and resulting distortion of the normal eye alignment. Although the red reflex appears normal bilaterally, retinoblastoma can still be present and affect one eye.

What is the gold standard imaging modality for evaluating pediatric brain tumors?

Explanation: MRI is the gold standard imaging modality for evaluating pediatric brain tumors. It provides detailed images of the brain's anatomy and allows for better characterization of the tumor's location, size, and surrounding structures. MRI can also aid in surgical planning and assessment of treatment response.

What is the first-line treatment for high-grade pediatric brain tumors?

Surgical resection followed by radiation therapyand chemotherapy.

Explanation: The first-line treatment for high-grade pediatric brain tumors, such as high-grade astrocytomas or medulloblastomas, typically involves surgical resection to remove as much of the tumor as possible. This is followed by adjuvant therapies such as radiation therapy, which targets remaining tumor cells, and chemotherapy, which helps to control tumor growth and prevent recurrence. The combination of surgery, radiation, and chemotherapy aims to maximize tumor control and improve the chances of long-term survival.

What is hemophilia?

Hemophilia is an inherited bleeding disorder characterized by a deficiency or dysfunction of clotting

Which clotting factor is deficient in hemophilia A?

factors, primarily factor VIII (hemophilia A) or factor IX (hemophilia B).

Hemophilia A is characterized by a deficiency of factor VIII.

Explanation: Factor VIII is essential for normal blood clotting, and its deficiency leads to impaired clot formation and prolonged bleeding.

What is the inheritance pattern of hemophilia?

Hemophilia is an X-linked recessive disorder, meaning it is more common in males and is passed down from carrier females.

Explanation: The gene mutations causing hemophilia are located on the X chromosome. Males have one X chromosome, so a single copy of the mutated gene results in the disorder. Females have two X chromosomes, and carriers of the gene mutation may have milder symptoms or be asymptomatic.

What is the typical presentation of hemophilia?

Hemophilia presents with prolonged bleeding after injuries, spontaneous joint bleeds, easy bruising, and excessive bleeding following surgeries or dental procedures.

Explanation: The deficiency or dysfunction of clotting factors in hemophilia leads to impaired blood clotting, resulting in the characteristic bleeding symptoms.

What is the primary difference between Hemophilia A and Hemophilia B?

The primary difference lies in the deficient clotting factor. Hemophilia A is caused by a deficiency or dysfunction of factor VIII, while Hemophilia B is caused by a deficiency or dysfunction of factor IX.

How does the severity of Hemophilia A and Hemophilia B compare?

On average, Hemophilia A tends to be more severe than Hemophilia B. Severe hemophilia is associated with less than 1% of normal factor activity, while moderate hemophilia ranges from 1% to 5% of normal activity. Mild hemophilia has factor activity levels between 5% and 40% of normal.

What laboratory test is used to diagnose and classify the severity of hemophilia A or B?

The specific laboratory test used is the factor activity assay.

Explanation: The factor activity assay measures the activity level of factor VIII in hemophilia A or factor IX in hemophilia B. The results help determine the severity of the condition as mild, moderate, or severe based on the percentage of factor activity.

What is the treatment of choice for acute bleeding episodes in hemophilia?

The treatment of choice for acute bleeding episodes in hemophilia is replacement therapy with the deficient clotting factor.

Explanation: Replacement therapy involves infusing the missing clotting factor to restore normal blood clotting and control bleeding

A 30-year-old male presents with a history of recurrent episodes of prolonged bleeding following minor injuries. He reports easy bruising and occasional spontaneous joint swelling without any

The correct answer is: A) Hemophilia A.

Explanation:

known trauma. On physical examination, there are no signs of active bleeding, but there is tenderness and limited range of motion in the left knee joint. Laboratory results show a prolonged activated partial thromboplastin time (aPTT) and a reduced factor VIII activity level. What is the most likely diagnosis?
A) Hemophilia A
B) Hemophilia B
C) von Willebrand disease
D) Factor V Leiden mutation

Based on the clinical presentation of recurrent episodes of prolonged bleeding, easy bruising, and spontaneous joint swelling, along with the laboratory findings of prolonged aPTT and reduced factor VIII activity, the most likely diagnosis is Hemophilia A. Hemophilia A is characterized by a deficiency or dysfunction of factor VIII, leading to impaired clot formation and prolonged bleeding. Hemophilia B (Option B) is characterized by a deficiency or dysfunction of factor IX. Von Willebrand disease (Option C) can also present with similar symptoms, but it is typically associated with normal or reduced factor VIII activity and abnormal von Willebrand factor levels. Factor V Leiden mutation (Option D) is a genetic mutation that predisposes individuals to venous thromboembolism and is not associated with the symptoms described in this case.

LEAD POISONING

What is the primary source of lead exposure in pediatric patients?

The primary source of lead exposure in pediatric patients is through ingestion of lead-containing dust, paint, or soil.

Explanation: Children may ingest lead by touching contaminated surfaces and then putting their hands or objects into their mouths.

What are the common symptoms of lead poisoning in children?

Common symptoms of lead poisoning in children include developmental delays, learning difficulties, irritability, loss of appetite, abdominal pain, and anemia.

Explanation: Lead can interfere with the development of the nervous system and affect various organs, leading to a range of symptoms.

Which laboratory test is used to measure blood lead levels?

The laboratory test used to measure blood lead levels is the venous blood lead level test.

Explanation: Blood lead level is a crucial indicator of lead exposure and helps in diagnosing lead poisoning. The Centers for Disease Control and Prevention (CDC) sets guidelines for acceptable blood lead levels in children.

What is the most appropriate treatment for lead poisoning in pediatric patients?

The most appropriate treatment for lead poisoning is chelation therapy with medications such as succimer or dimercaptosuccinic acid (DMSA).

Explanation: Chelation therapy involves the administration of medications that bind to lead and facilitate its excretion from the body.

What is a common long-term consequence of lead poisoning in pediatric patients?

Neurological and cognitive impairments are common long-term consequences of lead poisoning in pediatric patients.

Explanation: Lead has neurotoxic effects, and prolonged exposure can lead to permanent brain

A 4-year-old child presents with irritability, developmental regression, and abdominal pain. Physical examination reveals a lead line on the gingival margin. The child lives in an older home with peeling paint. Laboratory results show an elevated blood lead level. Which of the following is the most appropriate next step in management?
A) Start chelation therapy with succimer immediately.
B) Educate the family on lead-safe practices and provide resources for home lead remediation.
C) Perform an abdominal X-ray to assess for lead-containing foreign bodies.
D) Refer the child to a neurologist for further evaluation of developmental regression.

damage, resulting in learning difficulties and developmental delays.
the correct answer is: B) Educate the family on lead-safe practices and provide resources for home lead remediation.

Explanation: Based on the clinical presentation of irritability, developmental regression, abdominal pain, and the presence of a lead line on the gingival margin, along with the history of living in an older home with peeling paint, lead poisoning is highly suspected. The most appropriate next step in management is to educate the family on lead-safe practices and provide resources for home lead remediation (Option B). This step involves identifying and addressing lead hazards in the environment, such as removing or covering peeling paint, and implementing measures to prevent further lead exposure. Chelation therapy (Option A) is indicated for significantly elevated blood lead levels or severe symptoms, but immediate initiation is not necessary in this scenario. Performing an abdominal X-ray (Option C) is not a priority in the management of lead poisoning, as the clinical presentation and history strongly support the diagnosis. Referring the child to a neurologist (Option D) may be considered if there are specific concerns related to neurological symptoms or if the child's condition worsens, but it is not the most appropriate next step at this point.

LEUKEMIA

What is leukemia?

Leukemia is a type of cancer that affects the bone marrow and blood, resulting in abnormal production of white blood cells.

What are the common symptoms of leukemia in pediatric patients?

Common symptoms of leukemia in pediatric patients include fatigue, pallor, easy bruising or bleeding, frequent infections, bone pain, and swollen lymph nodes.

Explanation: These symptoms arise due to the disruption of normal blood cell production and the infiltration of leukemia cells in various tissues.

Which type of leukemia is more common in pediatric patients?

Acute lymphoblastic leukemia (ALL) is more common in pediatric patients.

Explanation: ALL is the most common type of leukemia in children, comprising about 75-80% of pediatric leukemia cases.

What is the diagnostic test of choice for leukemia?

The bone marrow aspiration and biopsy is the diagnostic test of choice for leukemia.

Explanation: A bone marrow aspiration and biopsy involve the collection of a small sample of bone marrow and examination under a microscope to determine the presence of leukemia cells and their characteristics.

What is the initial treatment approach for pediatric leukemia?	The initial treatment approach for pediatric leukemia typically involves a combination of chemotherapy.
	Explanation: Chemotherapy is the mainstay of treatment for pediatric leukemia. It aims to eliminate leukemia cells and induce remission.
Which type of leukemia is associated with a genetic abnormality called the Philadelphia chromosome?	Chronic Myeloid Leukemia (CML) is associated with the Philadelphia chromosome.
	Explanation: The Philadelphia chromosome results from a reciprocal translocation between chromosomes 9 and 22, leading to the formation of the BCR-ABL fusion gene, a hallmark of CML.
Which type of leukemia is most commonly seen in children?	Acute Lymphoblastic Leukemia (ALL) is the most common type of leukemia in children.
Which type of leukemia is characterized by the proliferation of immature myeloid cells in the bone marrow?	Acute Myeloid Leukemia (AML) is characterized by the proliferation of immature myeloid cells in the bone marrow.
Which type of leukemia is more commonly seen in older adults?	Chronic Lymphocytic Leukemia (CLL) is more commonly seen in older adults.
Which type of leukemia is characterized by the presence of Auer rods in the cytoplasm of leukemic blasts?	Acute Myeloid Leukemia (AML) is characterized by the presence of Auer rods in the cytoplasm of leukemic blasts.
	Explanation: Auer rods are rod-shaped cytoplasmic inclusions composed of fused azurophilic granules and are pathognomonic for AML.
Which type of leukemia is characterized by the presence of high lymphocyte counts, smudge cells, and lymphadenopathy?	Chronic Lymphocytic Leukemia (CLL) is characterized by the presence of high lymphocyte counts, smudge cells, and lymphadenopathy.

LYMPHOMA

What are the two main categories of lymphoma?	The two main categories of lymphoma are Hodgkin lymphoma (HL) and non-Hodgkin lymphoma (NHL).
Which type of lymphoma is characterized by the presence of Reed-Sternberg cells?	Hodgkin lymphoma (HL) is characterized by the presence of Reed-Sternberg cells. Reed-Sternberg cells are large, abnormal cells found in the lymph nodes of patients with Hodgkin lymphoma.
Which type of lymphoma is more common in pediatric patients?	Non-Hodgkin lymphoma (NHL) is more common in pediatric patients compared to Hodgkin lymphoma.
What is the most common presenting symptom of lymphoma in pediatric patients?	Painless lymphadenopathy (enlarged lymph nodes) is the most common presenting symptom of lymphoma in pediatric patients.
What is the first-line treatment for Hodgkin lymphoma in pediatric patients?	The first-line treatment for Hodgkin lymphoma in pediatric patients is combination chemotherapy, often followed by radiation therapy.
	Explanation: The treatment approach for Hodgkin lymphoma typically involves a combination of chemotherapy and, in some cases, radiation therapy.

NEUTROPENIA

What is neutropenia?	Neutropenia is a condition characterized by a decreased absolute neutrophil count (ANC) below 1000 cells/mm³.

What is the recommended diagnostic test for febrile neutropenia in pediatric patients?

Blood cultures are the recommended diagnostic test for febrile neutropenia in pediatric patients.

Explanation: Blood cultures help identify the causative organism and guide appropriate antibiotic therapy.

Which type of imaging may be indicated in febrile neutropenia to assess for suspected infections?

Imaging modalities such as chest X-ray or computed tomography (CT) may be indicated in febrile neutropenia to assess for suspected infections.

Explanation: Imaging can help identify pulmonary infiltrates, abscesses, or other sites of infection that may require further evaluation or intervention.

What is the treatment for neutropenia?

The commonly used antibiotic regimens for febrile neutropenia in pediatric patients include:

Antipseudomonal β-lactam (such as ceftazidime, cefepime, or meropenem) plus an aminoglycoside (such as gentamicin or amikacin): This combination provides coverage against both gram-negative bacteria, including Pseudomonas aeruginosa, and some gram-positive organisms.

Antipseudomonal β-lactam (such as ceftazidime, cefepime, or meropenem) plus vancomycin: This combination covers gram-negative bacteria, including Pseudomonas aeruginosa, and provides additional coverage against gram-positive organisms, including methicillin-resistant Staphylococcus aureus (MRSA).

Monotherapy with broad-spectrum β-lactam antibiotics (such as piperacillin-tazobactam): This regimen provides coverage against a wide range of gram-negative and gram-positive organisms and may be considered in low-risk patients or when the risk of resistant pathogens is low.

CRYPTORCHIDISM

When do the testes typically descend?	Spontaneous descent by 4-6 months old
Cryptorchidism increases the risk for what disease?	Testicular cancer
What are the signs and symptoms for cryptorchidism?	One or both testes absent from the scrotum at birth
What is the most common physical finding in a patient with cryptorchidism? **a) Absent testis** **b) Enlarged testis** **c) Empty scrotum** **d) Palpable testis in the inguinal canal**	Answer: d) Palpable testis in the inguinal canal Explanation: In cryptorchidism, the most common physical finding is a palpable testis in the inguinal canal. The testis may be located in the inguinal canal or higher in the abdomen. An absent testis or an empty scrotum suggests an undescended testis that cannot be palpated.

CYSTITIS

What is cystitis?	Cystitis refers to inflammation of the bladder, typically caused by a urinary tract infection (UTI). Explanation: Cystitis is a common condition characterized by inflammation of the bladder, usually resulting from a bacterial infection ascending from the urethra. It commonly presents with symptoms such as dysuria (painful urination), frequency, urgency, and sometimes hematuria (blood in the urine).
What is the most common cause of cystitis in the pediatric population?	E. Coli
Which diagnostic test should be performed in pediatric patients with recurrent cystitis? **a) Urine culture and sensitivity** **b) Voiding cystourethrogram (VCUG)** **c) Renal ultrasound** **d) Magnetic resonance imaging (MRI)**	Answer: a) Urine culture and sensitivity Explanation: In pediatric patients with recurrent cystitis, a urine culture and sensitivity should be performed. This test helps identify the causative pathogen and determine the appropriate antibiotic therapy. It can also detect antibiotic resistance, which is essential in cases of recurrent or persistent infections.
What is the treatment of choice for outpatient patients with cystitis?	Second or third-generation cephalosporin (e.g., cefdinir, cefpodoxime, cefotaxime)
What is the most common fungal pathogen of a UTI?	Candida albicans

ENURESIS

What is enuresis?	Involuntary urination (e.g., during the day or bedwetting at night) in children >5 years old
What is the workup for enuresis?	A thorough history, including recent history of voiding patterns, psychological stressors, emotional status, diet, hx or symptoms of DM, sleep patterns, fluid intake, or other causes that may be the origin of the voiding. Order UA, possible culture, +/- u/s of the bladder
What is the best initial for enuresis with no suspicion for pathological causes?	**First-line—behavior strategies with positive reinforcement** (do NOT make the patient feel bad for

wetting themselves), voiding diary, patient education (e.g., no drinking fluids before bed, good sleep routine hygiene), alarm devices

What is the drug of choice for enuresis? — Desmopressin

GLOMERULONEPHRITIS

What is the classic presentation for glomerulonephritis? — HTN, edema, and proteinuria

Which kind of casts are seen in glomerulonephritis? — RBC casts

What is the treatment for glomerulonephritis? — High dose corticosteroids

HYDROCELE

What is a hydrocele? — Peritoneal fluid build up between the tunica vaginalis layers

Which physical exam test confirms hydrocele? — Fluid around testicle that transilluminates
Can also perform u/s to check contents and ensure blood flow

What is the definitive treatment for a hydrocele that persists beyond the first year of life or causes significant discomfort?
a) Observation
b) Scrotal exploration and repair
c) Antibiotic therapy
d) Testicular aspiration

b) Scrotal exploration and repair

Explanation:
The definitive treatment for a hydrocele that persists beyond the first year of life or causes significant discomfort is scrotal exploration and repair. Surgical intervention, such as hydrocelectomy, is performed to remove or obliterate the hydrocele sac and prevent re-accumulation of fluid. This procedure is typically reserved for cases where the hydrocele does not resolve on its own or causes significant symptoms or cosmetic concerns.

HYPOSPADIAS

What is hypospadias? — Urethral meatus located on the ventral surface of the penis

Which is more common, hypospadias or epispadias? — Hypospadias is more common than epispadias

What is the recommended treatment for hypospadias?
a) Hormonal therapy with testostcronc
b) Observation and supportive care
c) Surgical repair
d) Antibiotic prophylaxis

c) Surgical repair

Explanation:
The recommended treatment for hypospadias is surgical repair. The goal of surgery is to reconstruct the urethra and relocate the urinarymeatus to the tip of the penis. The specific surgical technique and timing of the procedure depend on the severity of the hypospadias, age of the patient, and individual factors. Surgical repair is typically performed during early childhood to optimize functional and cosmetic outcomes.

What is the treatment for hypospadias? — Surgical management between the age of 6 months to 18 months of life. Refer our to urology for management

PARAPHIMOSIS

What is paraphimosis? — Retracted foreskin of an uncircumcised male cannot be returned to its normal anatomical position. Considered a medical emergency

What is the pathophysiology of paraphimosis?	Retracted foreskin is trapped posterior to the corona of the glans penis; forms a tight ring constricting the penile tissues, causing venous congestion, and potentially arterial occlusion
What are the signs and symptoms of paraphimosis?	Tenderness, erythematous, edematous; look for more troublesome signs (e.g., tight skin ring causes venous congestion), look for arterial occlusion and necrosis
What is the treatment for paraphimosis?	Manually retract the foreskin, cool compress. Definitive management—surgical incision under local anesthesia

PHIMOSIS

What is phimosis?	Inability to retract the foreskin over the head of the penis
Is phimosis considered a medical emergency?	No, paraphimosis is considered a medical emergency
What is the treatment for phimosis?	If asymptomatic, watch and wait, proper hygiene, stretching foreskin exercises, potential topical corticosteroid course for 4-8 weeks. If symptomatic, refer out for potential surgery (definitive)
Which of the following treatment options is typically considered when conservative management fails for pathological phimosis? **a) Topical corticosteroid cream** **b) Antibiotic therapy** **c) Circumcision** **d) Foreskin stretching exercises**	c) Circumcision Explanation: When conservative management fails for pathological phimosis, circumcision is often considered as a treatment option. Circumcision involves surgical removal of the foreskin, providing a permanent solution for the condition. It may be recommended in cases of severe or recurrent phimosis that do not respond to conservative measures.

TESTICULAR TORSION

What is testicular torsion?	Twisting of the spermatic cord
Which physical exams tests are performed for testicular torsion?	Absent cremasteric reflex and (-) Phren sign
What is the best test to order for testicular torsion?	U/s
What is the treatment for testicular torsion	Manual detorsion. If unable, urgent urology consult for orchiopexy (detorsion must occur within 4-6 hours)

VESICOURETERAL REFLUX

What is vesicoureteral reflux?	Retrograde flow of urine from the bladder into the ureter
What are signs and symptoms of vesicoureteral reflux?	Recurrent febrile urinary tract infections
Which diagnostic test is considered the gold standard for the diagnosis of vesicoureteral reflux? **a) Voiding cystourethrogram (VCUG)** **b) Renal ultrasound** **c) Magnetic resonance imaging (MRI)** **d) Urine culture**	a) Voiding cystourethrogram (VCUG) Explanation: Voiding cystourethrogram (VCUG) is considered the gold standard diagnostic test for vesicoureteral reflux. During a VCUG, contrast dye is instilled into the bladder, and X-ray images are taken during voiding to assess the presence and severity of reflux. VCUG provides important information about the anatomy and function of the urinary system, including the presence of VUR and any associated abnormalities.

What is the primary goal of treatment for vesicoureteral reflux?
a) Elimination of urinary tract infections (UTIs)
b) Restoration of normal kidney function
c) Prevention of bladder dysfunction
d) Correction of urinary incontinence

a) Elimination of urinary tract infections (UTIs)

Explanation:
The primary goal of treatment for vesicoureteral reflux is the elimination of urinary tract infections (UTIs). VUR increases the risk of UTIs, which can lead to kidney damage if left untreated. The management approach aims to prevent recurrent infections and minimize the potential for kidney injury. Treatment options may include antibiotic prophylaxis, surgical intervention, or a combination of both, depending on the severity of reflux and associated risks.

1. **A 12-year-old boy presents to the pediatrician for itchiness for three weeks. On exam, he has lichenified plaques and pruritus of the flexor surfaces, worse at the popliteal and antecubital fossae. Which of the following is the most likely diagnosis?**

   A) **Atopic dermatitis**
   B) **Psoriasis**
   C) **Contact dermatitis**
   D) **Seborrheic dermatitis**

A) Atopic dermatitis

Explanation:
The most likely diagnosis for this child with a pruritic rash on the flexural areas of the elbows and knees, erythematous scaly patches, excoriations, and lichenification is atopic dermatitis. Atopic dermatitis is a common chronic inflammatory skin condition characterized by pruritus, eczematous lesions, and a typical distribution pattern involving flexural areas in children.

B) Psoriasis typically presents with well-demarcated, erythematous plaques with thick, silvery-white scale. It commonly involves extensor surfaces such as the elbows and knees, but the description of excoriations and lichenification is more consistent with atopic dermatitis.

C) Contact dermatitis can cause an erythematous rash with pruritus but is usually localized to the site of contact with the allergen or irritant. The distribution and chronicity of the rash in this case make atopic dermatitis more likely.

D) Seborrheic dermatitis typically affects areas rich in sebaceous glands, such as the scalp, face, and central chest. It presents with erythematous plaques covered with greasy yellow scale. The distribution and chronicity of the rash described in this case make atopic dermatitis a more likely diagnosis.

2. **A 6-year-old male patient presents with recurrent episodes of abdominal pain and bloating. He also complains of diarrhea alternating with constipation. On physical examination, there is tenderness in the right lower quadrant. A complete blood count reveals an elevated eosinophil count. Which of the following is the most likely diagnosis?**

   A) **Irritable bowel syndrome (IBS)**
   B) **Crohn's disease**
   C) **Intussusception**
   D) **D) Eosinophilic gastroenteritis**

Answer: D) Eosinophilic gastroenteritis

Explanation:

The most likely diagnosis for this patient with recurrent abdominal pain, bloating, diarrhea alternating with constipation, tenderness in the right lower quadrant, and elevated eosinophil count is eosinophilic gastroenteritis. Eosinophilic gastroenteritis is an inflammatory condition of the gastrointestinal tract characterized by eosinophilic infiltration.

A) Irritable bowel syndrome (IBS) may present with similar symptoms but typically does not involve eosinophilic infiltration.

B) Crohn's disease is a chronic inflammatory bowel disease that can cause abdominal pain, diarrhea, and tenderness. However, the elevated eosinophil count in

3. **A 9-month-old irritable boy accompanied by his mother presents with a rash for ten days. The mother says he cries the most during diaper changes. She noticed his genital area becoming more red with "white flakes." On exam, he has an erythematous rash around the perianal and perineal areas with dull margins and satellite lesions. Which of the following is the best treatment of choice for your patient?**

A) **Hydrocortisone cream**
B) **Clotrimazole cream**
C) **Antibiotic ointment**
D) **Zinc oxide cream**

4. **A 3-year-old boy accompanied by his mother presents to the pediatrician for a rash for one week. He has a vesicular rash on his bilateral hands and feet with vesiculo-ulcerative lesions of the posterior pharynx. Which of the following etiologies most accurately characterizes the presumed diagnosis?**

A) **Coxsackievirus**
B) **Adenovirus**
C) **Rhinovirus**
D) **Varicella**
E) **Measles**

5. **Which of the following diagnoses is suggested by the presence of parotid gland swelling,**

this case suggests eosinophilic gastroenteritis as the more likely diagnosis.

C) Intussusception typically presents with sudden-onset severe abdominal pain, vomiting, and a palpable sausage-shaped mass. It is less likely in this case due to the chronicity of symptoms and the absence of typical findings.
Answer: B) Clotrimazole cream

The presented clinical scenario is suggestive of a Candidal diaper dermatitis, which is a fungal infection commonly seen in infants. The characteristic findings include an erythematous rash with dull margins and satellite lesions in the perianal and perineal areas. The treatment of choice for Candidal diaper dermatitis is an antifungal cream. Clotrimazole cream is an appropriate choice as it effectively treats yeast infections. Hydrocortisone cream, an anti-inflammatory steroid, may be used in certain cases, but it is not the primary treatment for fungal infections. Antibiotic ointment is not effective against yeast and may even exacerbate fungal infections. Zinc oxide cream is typically used for diaper rash caused by moisture or irritation but is not effective against fungal infections like Candida.
The correct answer is A) Coxsackievirus

Hand, Foot, and Mouth Disease (HFMD) is primarily caused by the Coxsackievirus, specifically the Coxsackievirus A16. It is a highly contagious viral infection that commonly affects young children. The characteristic presentation includes a vesicular rash on the hands, feet, and mouth, particularly the posterior pharynx. Other symptoms may include fever, sore throat, and malaise. HFMD is typically a self-limiting condition that resolves within a week or two.

Incorrect options:
B) Adenovirus: Adenovirus can cause various respiratory and gastrointestinal infections but is not the primary etiology for Hand, Foot, and Mouth Disease.
C) Rhinovirus: Rhinovirus primarily causes the common cold and is not associated with the specific vesicular rash seen in HFMD.
D) Varicella: Varicella, or chickenpox, is caused by the varicella-zoster virus and presents with a generalized vesicular rash, not limited to the hands, feet, and mouth.
E) Measles: Measles is caused by the measles virus and presents with a characteristic maculopapular rash that starts on the face and spreads to the rest of the body, which is different from the vesicular rash seen in HFMD.
Answer: A) Mumps

orchitis, and pancreatitis as a triad of symptoms?

A) Mumps
B) Orchitis
C) Pancreatic cancer
D) Testicular cancer
E) Sjögren's syndrome

Explanation: The presented triad of parotid gland swelling, orchitis, and pancreatitis is highly characteristic of mumps, a viral infection caused by the mumps virus. Mumps primarily affects the salivary glands, resulting in parotid gland swelling. It can also involve other organs, leading to orchitis (inflammation of the testicles) and pancreatitis (inflammation of the pancreas). Mumps is a highly contagious viral infection, and the symptoms can overlap with other conditions. However, the specific triad described in the question is most indicative of mumps.

Incorrect options:
B) Orchitis: Orchitis refers to inflammation of the testicles and can be a symptom of mumps, but it does not explain the presence of parotid gland swelling and pancreatitis in the presented triad.
C) Pancreatic cancer: Pancreatic cancer can cause pancreatitis, but it does not typically present with parotid gland swelling or orchitis.
D) Testicular cancer: Testicular cancer can cause orchitis-like symptoms, but it does not explain the presence of parotid gland swelling and pancreatitis in the presented triad.
E) Sjögren's syndrome: Sjögren's syndrome is an autoimmune condition characterized by dry eyes and dry mouth, but it does not typically cause parotid gland swelling, orchitis, or pancreatitis.

6. A 3-year-old child presents with fever, sore throat, and enlarged tonsils with exudates. On physical examination, there are palpable tender anterior cervical lymph nodes. A rapid antigen detection test for group A Streptococcus (GAS) is positive. Which of the following is the most appropriate next step in management?

A) Oral amoxicillin
B) Intramuscular penicillin G
C) Observation and supportive care
D) Azithromycin

Answer: B) Intramuscular penicillin G

Explanation:
The most appropriate next step in management for this child with fever, sore throat, enlarged tonsils with exudates, palpable tender anterior cervical lymph nodes, positive GAS rapid antigen test, and a confirmed diagnosis of streptococcal pharyngitis is intramuscular penicillin G. Intramuscular penicillin G is the treatment of choice for GAS pharyngitis in children.

A) Oral amoxicillin is an alternative treatment option for GAS pharyngitis. However, the intramuscular route is preferred for the initial treatment.
C) Observation and supportive care alone are not appropriate in the treatment of confirmed GAS pharyngitis.
D) Azithromycin is an alternative treatment for patients with penicillin allergy. However, in this case, the patient does not have a documented penicillin allergy, making penicillin G the preferred choice.

7. 5-year-old unvaccinated girl from Yemen presents with high fever, prodrome of cough, coryza, and conjunctivitis. The rash spreads in a cephalocaudal pattern, which of the following is the most likely diagnosis?

The correct answer is B) Measles

Explanation: Measles, also known as rubeola, is a highly contagious viral infection caused by the measles virus. The prodromal phase is characterized by symptoms such as high fever, cough, coryza (runny nose), and

A) German measles
B) Measles
C) Roseola
D) Erythema infectiosum
E) Hand-foot-mouth disease

8. **A 17-year-old girl presents with a vesicular genital rash for three days. She has a significant past medical history for recurrent HSV. The rash is painful and isolated to her trunk and extremities. Examination of the skin reveals many purple papules and macules with a dusky center surrounded by a light ring. She has a negative Nikolsky sign. Which of the following is the most likely diagnosis?**

A) Urticaria
B) Steven-Johnson syndrome
C) Erythema multiforme
D) Eczema herpeticum

9. **A 4-year-old girl presents to the pediatrician accompanied by his mother for facial "crusting" for two days. On exam, he is afebrile and in no acute distress. He has no known past medical history or allergies. Examination of the skin reveals a red rash with honey-colored crusts on the chin. She notes the rash is extremely itchy. Which of the following is the best initial treatment of choice?**

A) Cephalexin by mouth for seven days
B) Topical nystatin for five days
C) Erythromycin by mouth for seven days
D) Topical mupirocin for five days

conjunctivitis (pink eye). These symptoms are followed by the characteristic rash, which typically starts on the face and spreads downward in a cephalocaudal (head to toe) pattern.

German measles (Rubella) is a separate viral infection that presents with a milder rash and is usually associated with milder symptoms. Roseola is characterized by high fever followed by a rash, but the rash does not typically follow a cephalocaudal pattern. Erythema infectiosum (Fifth disease) presents with a slapped-cheek rash but does not typically have the same prodrome of symptoms. Hand-foot-mouth disease primarily affects the hands, feet, and mouth and is not associated with a cephalocaudal rash spreading pattern.

C) Erythema multiforme

Explanation: Erythema multiforme (EM) is a skin condition characterized by the presence of papules, macules, or vesicles with target-like or "iris" lesions. The lesions typically have a dusky center surrounded by a light ring, giving them a distinctive appearance. EM can be triggered by various factors, including infections, medications, and underlying herpes simplex virus (HSV) infections.

In this case, the patient's history of recurrent HSV and the characteristic skin findings, along with the presentation of painful vesicular rash on the trunk and extremities, are highly suggestive of erythema multiforme. Eczema herpeticum is a more extensive and severe HSV infection that typically occurs in patients with underlying atopic dermatitis and presents with widespread vesicular lesions. Steven-Johnson syndrome and urticaria would typically have different clinical manifestations and do not match the specific findings described in the scenario.

D) Topical mupirocin for five days

Explanation: The described clinical features are consistent with impetigo, a common bacterial skin infection that is often caused by Staphylococcus aureus or Streptococcus pyogenes. The honey-colored crusts are characteristic of impetigo. Treatment for localized impetigo typically involves topical antibiotics. Mupirocin is a commonly used topical antibiotic that is effective against the bacteria commonly associated with impetigo.

Incorrect options:
A) Cephalexin by mouth for seven days: Oral antibiotics may be required for more extensive or severe cases of

10. **A 12-year-old boy presents with a runny nose and sneezing for three weeks. He denies any fever, nausea, vomiting, diarrhea, shortness of breath or wheezing. On exam, his nares are patent with edematous nasal turbinates that are pale. Oropharynx is clear with no exudate or tonsillitis. Lungs are clear to auscultation bilaterally. Which of the following additional physical exam findings is likely to be found based on the presumed diagnosis?**

A) **Green discharge in the eyelids bilaterally**
B) **Swollen dark circles under the eyes bilaterally**
C) **Expiratory wheezing on auscultation of lungs bilaterally**
D) **Tympanic membrane bulging bilaterally**

11. **A 3-year-old child presents to the emergency department with sudden onset coughing and wheezing. The child's parent reports that the symptoms started immediately after the child was playing with small toy parts. On examination, the child has limited chest expansion on the right side, diminished breath sounds on the right, and persistent wheezing. Which of the following is the most likely diagnosis?**

A) **Asthma exacerbation**
B) **Pneumonia**
C) **Foreign body aspiration**
D) **Bronchiolitis**

impetigo, but for the presented scenario, topical treatment is the initial preferred choice.
B) Topical nystatin for five days: Nystatin is an antifungal medication used to treat fungal infections. It is not effective against bacterial infections such as impetigo.
C) Erythromycin by mouth for seven days: While erythromycin is an antibiotic effective against certain bacteria, it is not the first-line treatment for localized impetigo. Topical antibiotics are generally preferred for localized cases.
B) Swollen dark circles under the eyes bilaterally
Explanation: Green discharge in the eyelids bilaterally is characteristic of bacterial conjunctivitis. Expiratory wheezing on auscultation of lungs bilaterally is characteristic of an acute asthma exacerbation. Tympanic membrane bulging bilaterally is characteristic of acute otitis media.

Answer: C) Foreign body aspiration

Explanation: The clinical presentation of sudden onset coughing, wheezing, limited chest expansion on one side, diminished breath sounds, and a history of playing with small toy parts raises the suspicion of foreign body aspiration. In young children, foreign body aspiration occurs when an object becomes lodged in the airway, leading to partial or complete obstruction. Wheezing can occur due to airway narrowing caused by the presence of the foreign body. Diminished breath sounds can be attributed to reduced airflow in the affected lung.

Incorrect options:
A) Asthma exacerbation: While wheezing can be seen in both foreign body aspiration and asthma, the sudden onset of symptoms after a specific event and the findings of limited chest expansion and diminished breath sounds suggest a foreign body aspiration rather than an asthma exacerbation.
B) Pneumonia: Pneumonia may present with cough and wheezing, but it is less likely to cause limited chest expansion, diminished breath sounds, and sudden onset symptoms immediately after a specific event like playing with small toy parts.
D) Bronchiolitis: Bronchiolitis typically presents with cough, wheezing, and respiratory distress in infants and

12. **A 25-year-old patient presents with 4 days of acute upper respiratory tract infection, chills, coryza, and cervical lymphadenopathy. The most likely viral infection responsible for these symptoms is which of the following?**

A) **Influenza**
B) **Rhinovirus**
C) **Adenovirus**
D) **Respiratory syncytial virus (RSV)**

young children. However, it is less likely to cause limited chest expansion on one side and diminished breath sounds, as seen in this scenario.
Answer: A) Influenza

Explanation: The combination of symptoms, including acute upper respiratory tract infection, chills, coryza (nasal congestion), and cervical lymphadenopathy, is suggestive of influenza. Influenza is a viral respiratory infection that commonly presents with these symptoms. Chills and systemic symptoms are often seen in influenza, and cervical lymphadenopathy can occur due to immune responses in the lymph nodes.

Incorrect options:
B) Rhinovirus: Rhinovirus is a common cause of the common cold and can present with symptoms similar to influenza, but it typically does not cause significant chills or cervical lymphadenopathy.
C) Adenovirus: Adenovirus can cause respiratory tract infections and may lead to symptoms similar to influenza. However, the presence of cervical lymphadenopathy is less common with adenovirus infections.
D) Respiratory syncytial virus (RSV): RSV is a common cause of respiratory tract infections, especially in infants and young children. While it can present with upper respiratory symptoms, it is less likely to cause chills and cervical lymphadenopathy compared to influenza.
Answer: A) Croup

13. **A 2-year-old child presents to the pediatrician with a seal-like barking cough that has been worsening over the past 24 hours. The child's parent reports that the cough is most prominent at night and is associated with inspiratory stridor. On examination, the child appears otherwise well, with no signs of respiratory distress. Vitals show a heart rate of 110 beats per minute, respiratory rate of 24 breaths per minute, and oxygen saturation of 98% on room air. Which of the following is the most likely diagnosis?**

A) **Croup**
B) **Asthma**
C) **Pertussis**
D) **Epiglottitis**

Explanation: The clinical presentation of a 2-year-old child with a seal-like barking cough, worsening at night, inspiratory stridor, and otherwise well appearance is characteristic of croup, also known as laryngotracheobronchitis. Croup is a viral infection that causes inflammation of the upper airway, resulting in a distinctive cough that resembles a seal's bark. Inspiratory stridor, caused by narrowing of the airway, is often observed. The symptoms are typically worse at night and can be associated with a low-grade fever. The absence of significant respiratory distress and the vitals within normal range further support the diagnosis of croup in this case.

Incorrect options:
B) Asthma: Asthma typically presents with recurrent episodes of wheezing, shortness of breath, and chest tightness. While some children with asthma may have a cough, the seal-like barking cough and inspiratory stridor seen in this case are more characteristic of croup.
C) Pertussis: Pertussis, also known as whooping cough, can cause prolonged, paroxysmal coughing fits, often followed by a characteristic inspiratory whooping sound. The presentation in this case is more consistent

14. **What is the likely diagnosis for a patient who presents with a discrepancy in blood pressure between the left and right arms, along with a stronger radial pulse compared to the femoral pulse?**

A) **Coarctation of the Aorta**
B) **Aortic Stenosis**
C) **Aortic Dissection**
D) **Peripheral Arterial Disease (PAD)**

15. **What is the most common cause of pancreatitis in the pediatric population?**

A) **Measles**
B) **Mumps**
C) **Roseola**
D) **German measles**
E) **Fifth disease**

16. **A 12-month-old boy presents for a routine one-year visit. He is currently up to date on all**

with croup, as pertussis typically has different clinical features.

D) Epiglottitis: Epiglottitis is a rare, potentially life-threatening infection of the epiglottis. It typically presents with high fever, severe sore throat, drooling, and significant respiratory distress. The absence of respiratory distress and the more gradual onset of symptoms in this case make epiglottitis less likely. Coarctation of the aorta is a congenital heart defect characterized by a narrowing or constriction of the aorta, the main artery that carries oxygenated blood from the heart to the rest of the body. It often leads to a difference in blood pressure between the upper and lower extremities.

In this scenario, the presence of different blood pressure readings in the left and right arms suggests a significant pressure gradient across the narrowing in the aorta. The higher blood pressure in the arm (brachial blood pressure) compared to the leg (femoral blood pressure) is a classic finding in coarctation of the aorta. The radial pulse being stronger than the femoral pulse is another indicator of this condition.

Coarctation of the aorta can cause various symptoms, such as high blood pressure in the upper body and low blood pressure in the lower body, as well as leg fatigue or claudication (pain with exertion). It can also be associated with other congenital heart defects.

Confirmation of the diagnosis typically involves further evaluation with imaging studies such as echocardiography, magnetic resonance imaging (MRI), or computed tomography (CT) angiography.

Management of coarctation of the aorta usually involves surgical repair or catheter-based interventions to relieve the constriction and restore normal blood flow throughout the body. Prompt treatment is necessary to prevent complications and long-term cardiovascular issues.

B) Mumps

Explanation: Among the options provided, mumps is the most common cause of pancreatitis in the pediatric population. Mumps is a viral infection caused by the mumps virus, and it primarily affects the salivary glands. However, in some cases, mumps can lead to inflammation of the pancreas, resulting in pancreatitis.

While measles, roseola, German measles (rubella), and fifth disease (erythema infectiosum) are viral infections that can cause various symptoms, including rash, they are not commonly associated with pancreatitis.

The correct answer is B) atrial septal defect. Patency between the atrial septum. ASD is most common

of his immunizations. He has no past medical history recorded in the EMR. Upon exam, there is a wide, fixed S2 over the second left intercostal space. Which of the following is the most likely diagnosis?

A) Ventricular septal defect
B) Atrial septal defect
C) Tetralogy of Fallot
D) Coarctation of the aorta

congenital cardiac defect in patients with Down Syndrome. S/sx: mostly asymptomatic; incidental discover of heart murmur. If severe—respiratory tract infections, exertional dyspnea, or failure to thrive. PE: systolic ejection murmur. Wide, fixed S2 over the 2nd left ICS. Dx: CXR—cardiomegaly, pulmonary edema, right atrial enlargement. EKG—RAD, right ventricular hypertrophy. Transthoracic echo (TTE) is confirmatory. Tx: most resolve spontaneously. If severe—surgical patching

17. A 9-year-old boy presents to his pediatrician for right ear pain. He recently started his summer vacation and enjoys swimming at the local pool. On exam, his tympanic membranes are clear bilaterally with no bulging or effusion. The right external auditory canal is erythematous and edematous with malodorous discharge. Which of the following is the most likely etiology for the presumed diagnosis?

A) Haemophilus influenzae
B) Streptococcus pneumoniae
C) Pseudomonas aeruginosa
D) Streptococcus pyogenes
E) Moraxella catarrhalis

C) Pseudomonas aeruginosa is the correct answer

H flu, M. cat, strep pneumo, and strep pyogenes are commonly seen in acute otitis media. Et: swimmers, MC pathogen= pseudomonas aeruginosa. S/sx: ear pain, erythema, edema of ear canal. PE: thick purulent d/c in the external ear canal, pain when pulling ear. Treatment is topical fluroquinolone (e.g., ciprofloxacin)

18. A 12-year-old girl presents to the pediatrician for warts on her hand. Upon closer inspection, there are four 5cm cutaneous warts along the dorsal aspect of the third digit near the distal interphalangeal joint. There are no other skin lesions present elsewhere on the body. Which of the following medications is the treatment of choice?

A) Mupirocin
B) Nystatin
C) Salicylic acid
D) Clotrimazole

The correct answer is **C) salicylic acid**. Cutaneous warts are due to human papillomavirus. The diagnosis is made clinically. Most are self-resolving. Salicylic acid is considered first-line therapy. **A) Mupirocin** is the treatment of choice for impetigo. **B) nystatin** and C) **clotrimazole** are used for fungal causes such as tinea corporis

19. Which of the following accurately describes herpetic gingivostomatitis?

A) White plaques on buccal mucosa
B) Fever followed by mucosal purpuric lesions
C) Yellow ulcerative lesions
D) Flaccid bullae on a non-erythematous base

The correct answer is **C) yellow ulcerative lesions**. **A) white plaques on buccal mucosa** is characteristic of oral candidiasis. **B) fever followed by mucosal purpuric lesions** on the skin and mucous membranes is characteristic of Stevens-Johnson syndrome. **D) flaccid bullae on a non-erythematous base** is characteristic of bullous impetigo

20. A 4-year-old child presents with a 3-day history of acute otitis media. On examination, the tympanic membrane is erythematous and bulging. Which of the following is the most appropriate initial treatment?

Answer: B) Amoxicillin

Explanation:
The most appropriate initial treatment for this child with acute otitis media, erythematous and bulging tympanic membrane is amoxicillin. Amoxicillin is the first-line

A) **Observation and symptomatic care**
B) **Amoxicillin**
C) **Intramuscular ceftriaxone**
D) **Topical antibiotic ear drops**

antibiotic choice for the treatment of acute otitis media in children, unless there are specific indications for an alternative antibiotic.

A) Observation and symptomatic care alone are not appropriate for a child with acute otitis media and a bulging tympanic membrane.
C) Intramuscular ceftriaxone may be reserved for cases of treatment failure or severe illness.
D) Topical antibiotic ear drops are not the first-line treatment for acute otitis media. Systemic antibiotics are generally more effective in treating the infection.
The correct answer is D) mebendazole.
Pinworm infection # enterobiasis
- Et: enterobiasis vermicularis
- S/sx: perianal itching that is worse at night
- Dx: cellophane tape or scotch tape test
- Tx: **mebendazole** or albendazole

21. **A 2-year-old boy presents with perianal itching that is worse at night. A cellophane tape test is done in-office and under microscopy eggs are visualized. Which of the following is the most appropriate treatment?**

A) **Reassurance**
B) **Pyrantel pamoate**
C) **Hydrocortisone cream**
D) **Mebendazole**
E) **Cefepime**

22. **A 4-year-old boy accompanied by his mother presents to the emergency department with a cough that is worse at night for two days. The mother denies hoarseness or drooling. She endorses shortness of breath. He has no past medical history. He is not allergic to any medications. On exam, he is febrile with congestion and rhinorrhea. RR is 34 breaths per minute and oxygen saturation is 92%. On auscultation, there is inspiratory stridor. He has significant respiratory retractions along his thorax bilaterally and nasal flaring. Which of the following is the best initial step in the management?**

The correct answer is B) nebulized racemic epinephrine. When there are signs of respiratory distress (e.g., accessory muscle use, nasal flaring, cyanosis, > RR rate, grunting). Et: **most commonly viral, parainfluenza** being the most common virus. Bacterial causes include *S aureus, S. pneumo, H flu, and M. catarrhalis*
S/sx: seal-like barking cough, hoarseness, and inspiratory stridor
Dx: clinical diagnosis. CXR may identify subglottic narrowing (steeple sign)
Tx: immediate stabilization, support airway (supplemental oxygen, intubation). Mild to moderate—dexamethasone can reduce airway swelling within 6 hours. Moderate-severe—nebulized racemic epi

A) **Dexamethasone**
B) **Nebulized racemic epinephrine**
C) **Supplemental oxygen**
D) **Chest radiographs**

23. **A 3-year-old boy presents with a clonic-tonic seizure for six minutes and was rushed to the emergency department. Which of the following is the first-line therapy for status epilepticus?**

The correct answer is E) Lorazepam. A) Phenytoin, B) fosphenytoin, and C) valproic acid are considered second line and can be used if Lorazepam is unsuccessful. Ethambutol is first line for absence seizures.

A) **Phenytoin**
B) **Fosphenytoin**
C) **Valproic acid**
D) **Ethambutol**
E) **Lorazepam**

Explanation: Status epilepticus is a medical emergency characterized by prolonged or recurrent seizures that last for a significant duration without recovery. The immediate goal in managing status epilepticus is to promptly terminate the seizure activity to prevent complications and neurological damage. Lorazepam, a benzodiazepine, is considered the first-line therapy for status epilepticus.

Lorazepam is a rapid-acting anticonvulsant that can be administered intravenously or intramuscularly. It acts by enhancing the inhibitory effects of the neurotransmitter GABA, thus suppressing seizure activity. The recommended initial dose of lorazepam for the treatment of status epilepticus in children is typically 0.1 mg/kg, not exceeding 4 mg.

Phenytoin, fosphenytoin, and valproic acid are commonly used antiepileptic drugs, but they are not considered first-line therapies for acute seizure termination in status epilepticus. Ethambutol, on the other hand, is an antibiotic used in the treatment of tuberculosis and has no role in the management of status epilepticus.

24. A two-hour-old new-born infant boy is evaluated for cystic fibrosis. Sweat chloride testing shows evidence of disease and DNA testing is underway in the laboratory. Which of the following physical exam findings is likely to be found on exam?

A) Dullness to percussion
B) Increased tactile fremitus
C) Decreased thoracic cavity diameter
D) Nasal polyps
E) Decreased sputum

The correct answer is **D) nasal polyps**. Nasal polyps are a common finding in patients diagnosed with cystic fibrosis. **A) dullness to percussion** and **B) increased tactile fremitus** are findings seen in acute bacterial pneumonia. **C) decreased thoracic cavity diameter** is not seen in cystic fibrosis; in fact, increased anteroposterior thoracic cavity is increased. **E) decreased sputum** is incorrect; there is increased sputum production due to cystic fibrosis

25. A 16-year-old girl presents to the pediatrician for a sore throat for five days. She is accompanied by her mother who says her daughter has been in bed more than usual and "doesn't want to do anything." The daughter endorses malaise, fatigue, and a persistent fever. She denies drooling, hoarseness, shortness of breath, abdominal pain, nausea, vomiting or diarrhea. Her temperature is 101F. On exam, her posterior oropharynx is erythematous with exudate and cervical lymphadenopathy. She has splenomegaly upon palpation of the left inferior costal margin. She has no rashes. Lungs are clear to auscultation bilaterally. Which of the following is the most appropriate clinical intervention for your patient?

A) Recommend continued bed rest for five days
B) Amoxicillin for ten days
C) Amoxicillin-clavulanate for seven days
D) Initiate anti-viral therapy for seven days
E) Recommend no contact sports for one month

The correct answer is E) recommend no contact sports for one month. The patient has infectious mononucleosis. Clinical manifestations include: fever, tonsillitis +/- exudate, posterior cervical lymphadenopathy, fatigue, malaise, +/- hepatosplenomegaly, and a rash if given amoxicillin to treat bacterial strep pharyngitis. Dx: monospot test (**heterophile agglutination test**)
Tx: Self-limiting, refrain from contact sports for 4 weeks after infection resolves (because of splenomegaly). Symptomatic treatment includes antipyretic and analgesic therapy

26. **A 16-month-old boy presents to the emergency department accompanied by his mother for fever and right ear pain for three days. He has been pulling at his ear for two days. He was recently treated for right acute otitis media two weeks ago but the mother endorsed using the medication only for three out of the recommended ten day course. His temperature today is 39C (102.2F). On exam, his right tympanic membrane is bulging with decreased mobility on air insufflation. The external auditory canal is erythematous. The auricle is protruding anteriorly. The posterior right ear is warm, red, and tender to palpation. Which of the following is the next best step in the management of your patient?**

A) **Oral antibiotic therapy**
B) **IV antibiotic therapy**
C) **IM antibiotic therapy**
D) **X-ray of the temporal skull**
E) **CT scan of the sinuses bilaterally**

The correct answer is **B) IV antibiotic therapy**. Fever, ear pain, auricle protruding forward, and tenderness/erythema/warmth to the mastoid area highly suggest an **acute mastoiditis** as a complication of an untreated **acute otitis media**. The infection has spread from the tympanic membrane area to the mastoid air cells, which is a medical emergency due to potential osteonecrosis of the temporal/occipital bone area. Treatment requires prompt IV antibiotic therapy (e.g., vancomycin) and surgical drainage of the mucopurulent material. Consult otolaryngology.

27. **A 6-month-old boy is brought to the pediatrician by his parents for his routine wellness exam and vaccinations. He is up to date on his vaccinations. He has no pertinent past medical history. He has no known drug allergies. On exam, an erythematous rash is seen in the diaper area. The mother endorses a three-day rash but did not find it to be concerning. Upon further examination, the rash is erythematous and diffuse over the perineal and perianal regions sparing the inguinal folds and thigh creases with no satellite lesions. Which of the following is the most appropriate therapy for this patient?**

A) **High-potency topical corticosteroid ointment**
B) **Clotrimazole oral**
C) **Nystatin cream**
D) **Zinc oxide paste**
E) **Neosporin ointment**

The correct answer is **D) zinc oxide paste**. The diagnosis is **diaper dermatitis** (irritant contact dermatitis). A low potency ointment can be given, but **A) a high potency ointment** is not indicated and should be avoided in the diaper area. **B) Oral clotrimazole** is not indicated for contact dermatitis or candida dermatitis. **C) Nystatin cream** is indicated if the diagnosis was candida dermatitis. **E) Neosporin ointment** can result in a bacterial superinfection with diaper dermatitis and is not recommended.

28. **A 2-week-old infant girl accompanied by her parents presents to the pediatrician to establish care. The birth was uncomplicated, the mother was 40 weeks' gestation, and delivered her baby girl at-home with the help of her family in a rural part of town. She had little to no prenatal care prior to this visit. The mother notes her daughter sleeps for most of the day and night with minimal crying. On exam, she is afebrile, respirations are 38**

The correct answer is **C) iodine deficiency**. The diagnosis is **congenital hypothyroidism**. **Signs and symptoms** include round face, lethargy, protruding tongue, hoarse cry, distended abdomen, dry skin, hypotonia, hypothermia, poor weight gain, poor feeding, and constipation. **Workup** includes the following tests: best initial test—serum TSH elevated. **Confirmatory**—low free T4. Serum thyroid antibody testing—thyroglobulin antibodies and thyroid peroxidase antibodies—detectable in majority of autoimmune

breaths/min, HR is 84 beats/min, O2 sat is
98%, and all other vitals are unremarkable.
On exam, she is jaundiced with cool, dry skin.
She has poor head control and an enlarged
tongue. The abdomen is protuberant. Reflexes
are delayed. Which of the following is likely
the cause of the patient's signs and symptoms?

A) Growth hormone deficiency
B) Growth hormone excess
C) Iodine deficiency
D) Iodine excess
E) Pituitary tumor

29. **A 12-year-old girl presents to the pediatrician
accompanied by her mother for "hair loss" for
three months. Her mood and affect were
pleasant and reports good grades and plenty of
friends through her local soccer team. Her diet
is unchanged and includes vegetables and lean
meats and brown rice. She exercises regularly.
Her periods started last year and are
consistent each month. She has a family
history for psoriasis, rheumatoid arthritis, and
thyroid disease. Her TSH came back within
normal limits. On exam, she is afebrile, with
moist mucous membranes and good skin
turgor. Her skin has no lesions, plaques, or
dryness. She has no peripheral edema. Her
lungs are clear to auscultation bilaterally and
her heart has normal S1 and S2 sounds with
no arrythmias or murmurs. The only
remarkable finding from the exam were
exclamation point hairs under the microscope.
Which of the following is the most likely
diagnosis?**

A) Androgenic alopecia
B) Tinea capitis
C) Alopecia areata
D) Kerion
E) Trichotillomania

30. **A 4-year-old is brought with no past medical
history to the pediatrician by his mother for
"coughing attacks" for three days. She denies
hoarseness or change in voice quality. She said
one week ago he developed a runny nose and
cough after starting school at a new preschool.
Hoping it would resolve, she gave Claritin,
motrin, and cough syrup. He is not up to date
on his vaccinations. The cough continued to
worsen. During the exam, he was coughing
repeatedly and vomited shortly after. He is
afebrile with a 99% oxygen saturation.
Spirometry is done during the visit and reveals**

hypothyroidism cases; TSH receptor antibodies
detectable in 20% of autoimmune hypothyroidism.
Since the patient had an at-home delivery with little to
no prenatal care, it is likely the patient did not have
newborn screening for congenital hypothyroidism
(typically a heel stick serum check). **Treatment**
includes levothyroxine.

The correct answer is C) Alopecia areata. Alopecia
areata is associated with history of autoimmune
disorders. On exam, look for exclamation point hairs
(e.g., short broken hairs; the proximal portion is
narrower than the distal portion) which is
pathognomonic. B) Tinea capitis and D) kerion likely
present with more patchy hair loss; kerion is a
manifestation of the tinea capitis that must be treated
with oral griseofulvin to resolve the fungal problem.
Exclamation point hairs is not characteristic for tinea
capitis or kerion. A) Androgenic alopecia is the most
common cause of hair loss in females; however, does
not present with exclamation point hairs. Also, it
typically affects females more so after menopause. E)
Trichotillomania is a Psych condition in which the
patient plucks hairs from the scalp; however, it does not
present as exclamation point hairs. Rather, it presents in
inconsistent and random patterns of varying length and
size.

The correct answer is **E) liquid azithromycin**. The
diagnosis is **Bordetella pertussis**. He is in the first
phase (of three) which includes coughing fits (and post-
tussive emesis). **A), B), and C)** would be indicated if
the patient had **Croup**. However, there is no mention of
a "seal-like barking cough," or any signs of
laryngotracheobronchitis (e.g., inspiratory stridor, nasal
flaring, chest retractions). **D)** would be the correct
answer if an **acute asthma exacerbation** was expected.
However, the FEV_1/FVC ratio was within normal limits.
You would suspect asthma if the FEV_1 was < 80% or if
the FEV_1/FVC was < 70%. The most likely presentation
if Bordetella pertussis is based on the coughing fits and

an FEV_1/FVC of 80%. Which of the following is the most appropriate therapy?

A) Dexamethasone
B) Nebulized epinephrine
C) Cannulated oxygen
D) Nebulized albuterol
E) Liquid azithromycin

the post-tussive emesis and the fact that the patient is not up to date on their immunizations. **Bordetella pertussis** is a vaccine-preventable disease. **Treatment of choice** for Bordetella pertussis is **liquid azithromycin PO** in the pediatric population.

31. **A 6-year-old girl is accompanied by her father presents to the emergency department for right elbow pain for three hours. The father reports he was swinging her by the arm with his wife at the park when suddenly they felt a pop and she experienced acute pain. On exam, her right arm is held in flexion and adduction and the forearm is pronated; she is bracing her arm against her chest with the support of her left hand. She is guarding and hesitant. Sensation is intact over the bilateral deltoid, first dorsal webspace, medial, lateral, volar, and dorsal surfaces of the forearm and hand. 2+ radial pulse bilaterally. Compartments are soft. Skin is intact with no lesions. Which of the following is the most appropriate next step in the management of your patient?**

A) Orthopedic consultation
B) Posterior long arm splint
C) Thumb spica splint
D) Hyperpronation of the elbow joint
E) Supination and extension of the elbow joint

The correct answer is **D) hyperpronation of the elbow joint**. The diagnosis is radial head subluxation (e.g., Nursemaid elbow). **A) orthopedic consultation** is not necessary for a routine radial head subluxation in the emergency department. Consider orthopedic consultation if unable to reduce. Order plain radiographs. **B) posterior long arm splint** and **C) thumb spica splint** are not indicated in the management of a radial head subluxation. **E) supination and extension** is not the appropriate way to reduce the elbow. In fact, it is recommended to supinate and flex the elbow to reduce the radial head subluxation. Can order x-ray. Tx= reduction of radial head subluxation and pain management.
•Et: commonly occurs among children after caregiver tugs on outstretched forearm (e.g., swinging child by the arm or pulling the child upwards rapidly)
•S/sx: pain, tenderness, limited ROM, guarding, arm held in flexion and pronation (e.g., inability to supinate forearm); patient will resist forearm.

32. **A 2-year-old child presents to the clinic for a follow-up visit. The child's immunization records show incomplete vaccinations. The parents report concerns about vaccine side effects. What is the most appropriate response by the healthcare provider?**

A) **Reassure the parents that vaccines are safe and effective and explain the importance of completing the child's vaccinations.**
B) **Respect the parents' concerns and recommend alternative approaches to prevent diseases.**
C) **Advise the parents to delay further vaccinations until the child is older.**
D) **Dismiss the parents' concerns and insist on completing the child's vaccinations immediately.**

Answer: A) Reassure the parents that vaccines are safe and effective and explain the importance of completing the child's vaccinations.

Explanation: It is important to address parental concerns regarding vaccine safety but also emphasize the safety and effectiveness of vaccines. Reassuring the parents and educating them about the benefits of vaccinations is the most appropriate response.

33. **At what age do most infants start to roll over from their back to their stomach?**

Answer: B) 4 months

A) 2 months
B) 4 months
C) 6 months
D) 8 months

Explanation: Most infants begin to roll over from their back to their stomach around 4 months of age. However, the timing can vary among individuals.

34. A 4-year-old boy presents to the clinic accompanied by his parents. They report concerns about his development, noting that he rarely makes eye contact, has delayed speech, and exhibits repetitive behaviors such as hand flapping. They also mention that he has difficulties with social interactions and does not respond to his name being called. Based on the patient's presentation, which disorder is most likely the cause of his symptoms?

A) Attention-Deficit/Hyperactivity Disorder (ADHD)
B) Generalized Anxiety Disorder (GAD)
C) Autism Spectrum Disorder (ASD)
D) Language Disorder

Explanation: C) Autism Spectrum Disorder (ASD). The patient's delayed speech, lack of eye contact, repetitive behaviors, and difficulties with social interactions are consistent with the diagnostic criteria for ASD.

35. A 16-year-old adolescent presents with episodes of sudden palpitations and a sensation of a racing heart. The episodes typically resolve spontaneously within a few minutes. An electrocardiogram (ECG) shows a regular narrow complex tachycardia with a ventricular rate of 200 beats per minute. Vagal maneuvers fail to terminate the tachycardia. Which of the following is the most appropriate initial treatment?

A) Adenosine
B) Synchronized cardioversion
C) Beta-blockers
D) Radiofrequency ablation

Answer: A) Adenosine

Explanation:
The most appropriate initial treatment for this adolescent with episodes of sudden palpitations, a sensation of a racing heart, a regular narrow complex tachycardia, and a ventricular rate of 200 beats per minute is adenosine. Adenosine is the treatment of choice for terminating supraventricular tachycardia (SVT) due to its ability to transiently interrupt the reentrant circuit responsible for the tachycardia.

B) Synchronized cardioversion is reserved for unstable patients or those with hemodynamic compromise, which is not the case in this scenario.
C) Beta-blockers can be used for long-term management and prevention of recurrent SVT. However, adenosine is the preferred initial treatment to acutely terminate the tachycardia.
D) Radiofrequency ablation may be considered for patients with recurrent or refractory SVT, but it is not the appropriate initial treatment choice in this case.

36. Which of the following is a hallmark symptom of Major Depressive Disorder (MDD)?

A) Grandiosity and inflated self-esteem
B) Racing thoughts and flight of ideas
C) Persistent low mood and anhedonia
D) Intense fear and panic attacks

Answer: C) Persistent low mood and anhedonia

Explanation: Persistent low mood, along with anhedonia (loss of interest or pleasure in activities), is a hallmark symptom of Major Depressive Disorder (MDD). These symptoms must be present for at least two weeks to meet the diagnostic criteria for MDD.

37. A 14-year-old male presents with progressive pain and swelling in his left leg. On physical examination, a palpable mass is noted on the

Explanation: The most likely diagnosis in this case is osteosarcoma (Option A). Osteosarcoma commonly affects the metaphysis of long bones and presents with

distal femur. Laboratory tests reveal elevated serum alkaline phosphatase levels. Radiographs show a destructive lesion with cortical destruction. What is the most likely diagnosis?

A) Osteosarcoma
B) Ewing sarcoma
C) Chondrosarcoma
D) Osteochondroma
E) Osteomyelitis

38. A 19-year-old female presents with a painless mass in her left thigh. On physical examination, a firm, immobile mass is palpated. Radiographs reveal a well-circumscribed, cortical-based lesion with a thin layer of reactive bone. What is the most likely diagnosis?

A) Osteosarcoma
B) Giant cell tumor
C) Ewing sarcoma
D) Chondrosarcoma
E) Osteochondroma

39. A 14-year-old male presents with a several-week history of pain and swelling in his right thigh. On physical examination, tenderness is noted over the affected area. Laboratory tests reveal an elevated erythrocyte sedimentation rate (ESR). Imaging shows a lytic lesion with periosteal reaction. What is the most appropriate next step in the diagnosis of this patient?

A) Fine-needle aspiration biopsy
B) Core needle biopsy
C) Surgical excisional biopsy
D) MRI of the affected area
E) Plain radiographs of the chest

40. Which of the following is the primary treatment modality for localized osteosarcoma?

A) Radiation therapy

pain, swelling, and a palpable mass. Elevated serum alkaline phosphatase levels are frequently observed in patients with osteosarcoma. Radiographic findings typically include a destructive lesion with cortical destruction, periosteal reaction, and soft tissue mass. Ewing sarcoma (Option B) may present similarly, but it is typically seen in younger patients and is associated with the presence of EWSR1 gene rearrangement. Chondrosarcoma (Option C) typically arises from the cartilage and presents as a slow-growing mass. Osteochondroma (Option D) is a benign bone tumor characterized by an overgrowth of cartilage-capped bone projecting from the surface. Osteomyelitis (Option E) is an infection of the bone, which may present with pain, swelling, and fever.

Explanation: The most likely diagnosis in this case is giant cell tumor (Option B). Giant cell tumors commonly occur in the epiphysis of long bones, particularly around the knee, and typically present as a painless mass. On physical examination, they are often firm and immobile. Radiographically, giant cell tumors are characterized by well-circumscribed, cortical-based lesions with a thin layer of reactive bone. Osteosarcoma (Option A) presents with a destructive lesion, not a well-circumscribed mass. Ewing sarcoma (Option C) typically presents with pain, swelling, and a soft tissue mass, and may have associated cortical destruction. Chondrosarcoma (Option D) typically arises from the cartilage and does not present as a cortical-based lesion. Osteochondroma (Option E) is a benign tumor with a characteristic bony outgrowth.

Explanation: The most appropriate next step in the diagnosis of this patient is core needle biopsy (Option B). Ewing sarcoma is a malignant bone tumor commonly seen in children and young adults. The classic radiographic findings include a lytic lesion with periosteal reaction. To confirm the diagnosis, a tissue sample should be obtained for histopathological examination. Core needle biopsy is the preferred method as it provides an adequate sample for diagnosis while minimizing the risk of tumor seeding. Fine-needle aspiration biopsy (Option A) may not provide enough tissue for a definitive diagnosis. Surgical excisional biopsy (Option C) is not typically performed for suspected Ewing sarcoma due to the risk of tumor dissemination. MRI (Option D) is useful for evaluating the extent of disease, but biopsy is required for a definitive diagnosis. Plain radiographs of the chest (Option E) are necessary to evaluate for the presence of pulmonary metastases, which are common in Ewing sarcoma, but biopsy should be performed first.

Explanation: The primary treatment modality for localized osteosarcoma is surgical resection (Option C). Surgical resection aims to remove the tumor with negative margins, along with the surrounding affected bone and soft tissues. Chemotherapy (Option B) is an

B) **Chemotherapy**
C) **Surgical resection**
D) **Targeted therapy**
E) **Hormone therapy**

integral part of osteosarcoma treatment and is typically administered before and after surgery. Radiation therapy (Option A) is not typically used as a primary treatment modality for osteosarcoma. Targeted therapy (Option D) may be used in certain cases where specific molecular targets are identified, but it is not the primary treatment. Hormone therapy (Option E) is not effective in the treatment of osteosarcoma.

Answer: C) Sulfonylureas

41. **Which medication class stimulates insulin release from pancreatic beta cells and may cause hypoglycemia?**

A) **Biguanides**
B) **GLP-1 receptor agonists**
C) **Sulfonylureas**
D) **SGLT-2 inhibitors**

Explanation: Sulfonylureas are a class of oral antidiabetic medications that work by stimulating insulin release from pancreatic beta cells. They act by closing ATP-sensitive potassium channels on the beta cell membrane, leading to depolarization and subsequent release of insulin. However, sulfonylureas can sometimes lead to hypoglycemia, particularly if taken in excessive doses or if meal timing is irregular.

Incorrect choices:
A) Biguanides, such as metformin, work by reducing glucose production in the liver and increasing insulin sensitivity in peripheral tissues. They do not directly stimulate insulin release from pancreatic beta cells and are not associated with an increased risk of hypoglycemia.
B) GLP-1 receptor agonists, such as exenatide and liraglutide, mimic the action of the hormone GLP-1 and promote insulin release, but they do not directly stimulate insulin release from pancreatic beta cells. They have a low risk of causing hypoglycemia.
D) SGLT-2 inhibitors, such as empagliflozin and dapagliflozin, work by inhibiting glucose reabsorption in the kidneys, leading to increased urinary glucose excretion. They do not directly stimulate insulin release from pancreatic beta cells and are not associated with an increased risk of hypoglycemia.

Answer: C) GLP-1RA mimics the effects of the hormone GLP-1 and promotes insulin release, inhibits glucagon secretion, slows gastric emptying, and promotes satiety.

42. **What is GLP-1 receptor agonist (GLP-1RA) and how does it work in diabetes management?**

A) **GLP-1RA is an oral antidiabetic medication that improves insulin sensitivity.**
B) **GLP-1RA is a class of medications used to treat type 1 diabetes.**
C) **GLP-1RA mimics the effects of the hormone GLP-1 and promotes insulin release, inhibits glucagon secretion, slows gastric emptying, and promotes satiety.**
D) **GLP-1RA is a long-acting basal insulin.**

Explanation: GLP-1 receptor agonists, such as exenatide and liraglutide, are injectable medications used in the treatment of type 2 diabetes. They work by mimicking the action of glucagon-like peptide 1 (GLP-1), a hormone that is released in response to food intake. GLP-1 receptor agonists enhance insulin secretion from pancreatic beta cells, inhibit glucagon secretion from alpha cells, slow down gastric emptying, and promote a feeling of fullness (satiety). These actions help lower blood glucose levels, promote weight loss, and improve overall glycemic control in individuals with type 2 diabetes.

Incorrect choices:

43. **What is the hallmark electrocardiogram (ECG) finding associated with severe hypercalcemia?**

A) **Prolonged QT interval**
B) **Peaked T waves**
C) **PR interval prolongation**
D) **QRS complex widening**

44. **Which of the following medications can contribute to the development of hypercalcemia?**

A) **Nonsteroidal anti-inflammatory drugs (NSAIDs)**
B) **Proton pump inhibitors (PPIs)**
C) **Beta-blockers**
D) **Statins**

45. **A 2-year-old child presents to the pediatrician with a complaint of a white reflection in the right eye noticed by the parents in flash photographs. On examination, the child's right**

A) GLP-1 receptor agonists are not oral medications but are administered via subcutaneous injection.
B) GLP-1 receptor agonists are primarily used in the treatment of type 2 diabetes, not type 1 diabetes.
D) GLP-1 receptor agonists are not forms of insulin but act as adjunctive therapies to improve glycemic control in individuals with type 2 diabetes.
A) Prolonged QT interval

Explanation: Severe hypercalcemia can have cardiac manifestations, including the prolongation of the QT interval on the electrocardiogram (ECG). The QT interval represents the time it takes for ventricular depolarization and repolarization. Prolonged QT interval increases the risk of ventricular arrhythmias, such as torsades de pointes. It is important to monitor and manage hypercalcemia promptly to prevent cardiac complications.

Incorrect choices:
B) Peaked T waves are typically associated with hyperkalemia, not hypercalcemia.
C) PR interval prolongation is often seen in conditions affecting the atrioventricular (AV) conduction, such as heart block, but is not a characteristic finding in hypercalcemia.
D) QRS complex widening is usually observed in conditions affecting the ventricular depolarization, such as bundle branch block, but is not a specific finding in hypercalcemia.
Answer: B) Proton pump inhibitors (PPIs)

Explanation: Proton pump inhibitors (PPIs) are commonly used to treat conditions such as gastroesophageal reflux disease (GERD) and peptic ulcers. Prolonged use of PPIs can lead to hypercalcemia by impairing calcium absorption in the intestines. This occurs due to reduced gastric acid production, which is necessary for calcium ionization and subsequent absorption.

Incorrect choices:
A) Nonsteroidal anti-inflammatory drugs (NSAIDs) can cause kidney-related complications, including acute kidney injury, but they do not directly contribute to hypercalcemia.
C) Beta-blockers primarily affect the cardiovascular system by reducing heart rate and blood pressure. They are not known to cause hypercalcemia.
D) Statins are medications used to lower cholesterol levels and have no direct association with hypercalcemia.
The most likely diagnosis in this patient is B) retinoblastoma.

pupil appears white, while the left eye appears normal. There are no other abnormal findings on physical examination. The child has no significant past medical history, and there is no family history of eye conditions or cancers. What is the most likely diagnosis?

A) Glaucoma
B) Retinoblastoma
C) Cataract
D) Strabismus

46. A 7-year-old male presents with symptoms of dysuria, frequency, and urgency for the past two days. He denies fever or abdominal pain. Physical examination reveals suprapubic tenderness. Urinalysis demonstrates pyuria and positive leukocyte esterase. What is the next best step in management?

A) Start empiric antibiotic therapy with trimethoprim-sulfamethoxazole (TMP-SMX)
B) Obtain a urine culture and sensitivity
C) Perform a renal ultrasound
D) Initiate intravenous antibiotics

Explanation: The presence of a white pupil (leukocoria) in flash photographs is a classic sign of retinoblastoma in young children. This abnormal reflection occurs due to the presence of a tumor in the retina, which interferes with the normal red reflex seen in healthy eyes. Retinoblastoma is a malignant tumor that arises from retinal cells and is the most common intraocular malignancy in children.

In this case, the unilateral involvement of the right eye suggests the possibility of a sporadic (non-hereditary) retinoblastoma. However, further evaluation, including a detailed ophthalmological examination, imaging studies (such as ocular ultrasound or MRI), and potentially genetic testing, would be necessary to confirm the diagnosis and determine the extent of the disease.

Prompt identification and management of retinoblastoma are crucial to prevent local invasion, metastasis, and preserve vision. Treatment options may include enucleation (removal of the affected eye) if the tumor is localized and advanced, or local therapies (such as laser therapy, cryotherapy, or plaque brachytherapy) if the tumor is confined to the eye and vision preservation is possible.

Answer:
b) Obtain a urine culture and sensitivity

Explanation:
The next best step in management is to obtain a urine culture and sensitivity. This is important to identify the causative organism and determine the most appropriate antibiotic therapy. While the clinical presentation and urinalysis findings suggest a urinary tract infection (UTI), confirming the diagnosis and selecting the most effective antibiotic should be based on the results of urine culture and sensitivity.

Incorrect options:
a) Start empiric antibiotic therapy with trimethoprim-sulfamethoxazole (TMP-SMX): This option is incorrect because although empiric antibiotic therapy is necessary for the treatment of UTI, it is important to obtain a urine culture and sensitivity before initiating antibiotics to guide appropriate therapy.
c) Perform a renal ultrasound: This option is incorrect because a renal ultrasound is not the immediate next step in the management of uncomplicated cystitis. Renal ultrasound is primarily indicated for evaluating structural abnormalities of the kidneys and urinary tract, and it may be considered in specific cases (e.g., recurrent infections, atypical presentations).
d) Initiate intravenous antibiotics: This option is incorrect because intravenous antibiotics are not typically required for the management of uncomplicated cystitis. Intravenous antibiotics are reserved for severe

47. **Which physical finding is characteristic of a hydrocele?**

A) **Transillumination**
B) **Absence of cremasteric reflex**
C) **Tender scrotum**
D) **Palpable scrotal mass**

infections, such as pyelonephritis, or cases where the patient cannot tolerate oral antibiotics.

Answer: a) Transillumination

Explanation:
Transillumination is a characteristic physical finding in a hydrocele. When a light source is shined through the scrotum, the fluid-filled sac appears as a uniformly illuminated, translucent mass. This helps differentiate a hydrocele from other scrotal conditions, such as a solid mass or hernia.

Incorrect options:
b) Absence of cremasteric reflex: This option is incorrect because the absence of the cremasteric reflex is not specific to a hydrocele. The cremasteric reflex involves the elevation of the testicle in response to stroking the inner thigh and is commonly absent in infants.
c) Tender scrotum: This option is incorrect because a hydrocele is typically painless and not associated with tenderness. Scrotal tenderness may indicate other conditions, such as epididymitis or testicular torsion.
d) Palpable scrotal mass: This option is incorrect because a hydrocele is a fluid-filled sac and may not be palpable as a distinct mass. However, a large hydrocele may cause scrotal enlargement or fullness.

Answer: A) Iron deficiency anemia

48. **A 19-year-old male patient presents with fatigue, dyspnea on exertion, and pale conjunctiva. Laboratory tests reveal a hemoglobin level of 8 g/dL, mean corpuscular volume (MCV) of 78 fL, and red blood cell (RBC) count of 3.5 million/mm³. Peripheral blood smear shows hypochromic and microcytic red blood cells with anisocytosis and poikilocytosis. Which of the following is the most likely diagnosis?**

A) **Iron deficiency anemia**
B) **Thalassemia**
C) **Vitamin B12 deficiency anemia**
D) **D) Anemia of chronic disease**

Explanation:
The most likely diagnosis for this patient with fatigue, dyspnea on exertion, pale conjunctiva, hemoglobin level of 8 g/dL, MCV of 78 fL, red blood cell count of 3.5 million/mm³, and hypochromic and microcytic red blood cells on peripheral blood smear is iron deficiency anemia. Iron deficiency anemia is the most common type of anemia and is characterized by decreased iron stores leading to insufficient production of hemoglobin and red blood cells.

B) Thalassemia is a genetic disorder that leads to abnormal hemoglobin production and can cause microcytic anemia. However, the absence of specific findings suggestive of thalassemia (such as target cells or nucleated red blood cells) and the low MCV in this case make iron deficiency anemia more likely.
C) Vitamin B12 deficiency anemia typically presents with macrocytic red blood cells (high MCV), and the peripheral blood smear findings in this case suggest microcytic red blood cells.
D) Anemia of chronic disease is characterized by normocytic or microcytic red blood cells, but it is typically associated with underlying chronic inflammatory conditions or malignancy. The low MCV and absence of specific findings suggestive of anemia of

49. **An 18-year-old female patient presents with fatigue, weight gain, constipation, and dry skin. On physical examination, her pulse is 55 bpm, blood pressure is 120/80 mmHg, and there is cool, dry skin. Laboratory tests reveal an elevated thyroid-stimulating hormone (TSH) level and low free thyroxine (FT4) level. Which of the following is the most appropriate next step in management?**

A) **Thyroid ultrasound**
B) **Levothyroxine therapy**
C) **Thyroid antibody testing**
D) **Thyrotropin-releasing hormone (TRH) stimulation test**

50. **A 16-year-old male patient presents with acute-onset severe pain in his right testicle. On physical examination, the right testicle is high-riding, tender, and horizontally positioned. The cremasteric reflex is absent. Which of the following is the most appropriate next step in management?**

A) **Doppler ultrasound of the scrotum**
B) **Manual detorsion of the testicle**
C) **Surgical exploration and orchiopexy**
D) **Analgesic medication and scrotal support**

chronic disease make iron deficiency anemia more likely.
Answer: B) Levothyroxine therapy

Explanation:
The most appropriate next step in management for this 35-year-old female patient with fatigue, weight gain, constipation, dry skin, bradycardia, elevated TSH level, and low FT4 level is levothyroxine therapy. These clinical and laboratory findings are consistent with hypothyroidism, and levothyroxine replacement is the treatment of choice.

A) Thyroid ultrasound may be performed to evaluate the thyroid gland's size, structure, and any nodules. However, in this case, the clinical presentation and laboratory findings are sufficient to make a diagnosis of hypothyroidism, and treatment initiation is warranted.
C) Thyroid antibody testing, such as anti-thyroid peroxidase (anti-TPO) antibodies, can be helpful in diagnosing autoimmune thyroid disorders such as Hashimoto's thyroiditis. However, the diagnosis of hypothyroidism can be made based on clinical and laboratory findings, and treatment initiation is the priority.
D) The TRH stimulation test is used in cases of suspected central hypothyroidism to assess the pituitary-thyroid axis. In primary hypothyroidism, like in this case, the TSH level is elevated, indicating a defect at the level of the thyroid gland itself. Treatment with levothyroxine is the appropriate next step.
Answer: C) Surgical exploration and orchiopexy

Explanation:
The most appropriate next step in management for this 16-year-old male patient with acute-onset severe testicular pain, high-riding tender testicle, horizontal position, and absent cremasteric reflex is surgical exploration and orchiopexy. Testicular torsion is a surgical emergency, and prompt intervention is necessary to salvage the testicle.

A) Doppler ultrasound of the scrotum can help confirm the diagnosis of testicular torsion by demonstrating absent or reduced blood flow. However, the definitive management is surgical exploration and orchiopexy.
B) Manual detorsion of the testicle may be attempted as a temporary measure to restore blood flow before definitive surgical intervention. However, it is not the definitive treatment.
D) Analgesic medication and scrotal support may provide temporary pain relief but do not address the underlying torsion and can lead to testicular loss if not promptly treated.

(Page intentionally left blank for students to leave notes here)